INTERMITTENT FASTING FOR WOMEN OVER 50

21 days to Reset Metabolism, Increase Energy, Detox Your Body For A Rapid Weight Loss & Delay Aging | 120 Healthy Recipes - Including Meal Plan

Adele Glenn

Table Of Contents

To you,

Helping to create the perfect you.

Introduction

Congratulations on downloading this book and thank you for doing so. This book will help you in understanding the concepts of intermittent fasting for women after 50.

Intermittent fasting is an amazing concept that has helped innumerable people in losing weight and their belly fat. However, the utility of intermittent fasting goes much beyond weight loss. It is a complete wellness concept. It can help you in complete healing of the body. It can help your body in correcting the problems that have been developing inside without symptoms.

It is an amazing concept and very easy to follow, it is not the same for men and women. Also most importan, it is not the same if you have 20 or 30 years old or if you are 50 or more years old. Don't worry, it is not more difficult, it is only different. Our bodies change their needs every age and we have to change our habits. There are some major things that make intermittent fasting for women after 50 and this book will bring them out for you.

This book contains two parts:

The first part
- will explain you what happens to your body during pre-menopause and menopause and why you can't wait to save your health.

- will explain the various intermittent fasting protocols in detail and help you in choosing the best fit for yourself.

- will explain in detail the things you need to keep in mind for making your weight loss goals successful. It will give you deep insights into weight loss and the way intermittent fasting can help in it.

- will give you expert tips and clear some of the misconceptions. It will explain the common mistake made by people that can stop their progress. It will also explain the ways in which you can remain motivated throughout your way.

In the second part:

- you will find what to do in practice
- you will learn the best of two plans when you use the intermittent fasting techniques, specifically the 16/8 plan.
- how to accelerate your weight loss
- More than 120 easy and tasty recipes to make your journey happy
- 21 day meal plan to help you organize your life

The main objective of this book is to be helpful in your weight loss goals through intermittent fasting.

There are plenty of books on this subject on the market, thanks again for choosing this one! Every effort was made to ensure it is full of as much useful information as possible, please enjoy!

Chapter 1:

The only thing you need: The Right Mindset

Changing your mentality about weight loss goes beyond feeling good; it's about the outcome. A study at the University of Syracuse indicates that the more unhappy women are with their bodies, the more likely they are to skip exercise. And just focusing on the fact that you're overweight is forecasting a potential weight gain – according to studies reported in the International Journal of Obesity in 2015.

It all starts With Your Mindset

Many people who are struggling to eat healthily have what researchers term a "closed mentality." These people believe that nothing can ever change, and they take this belief with them in beginning a new weight loss plan. They think that their health issues are simply the effects of poor biology or that the embarrassment of solving the problem would reverse any improvements.

For certain people with a fixed mentality, long before it begins, a change of diet is futile. In reality, many would prefer to stay obese because it feels safer and less stressful than attempting to make a change in lifestyle.

Unfortunately, anyone who wants to move to a healthier lifestyle without changing their attitude first will soon get discouraged. That's because the journey to a healthy lifestyle doesn't happen overnight. There are no magic foods, no matter what the magazine said or what some star did to shed baby weight or to dress for a new role.

A growth mindset is not a crazy dreamer mindset when it comes to goals. When setting your targets, always make sure that they are fair. Keep note of how many balanced meals you consume, relative to how many might not be. Act to increase the number of nutritious meals you consume each week.

You've got to understand more than anything that your mindset may be what held you off. The good news is that you're well on your way to make a meaningful difference when you know that mindset is part of the problem!

Steps you can take to change your mindset.

Adjust your Priorities

The reason might be to lose weight, but that should not be the target. Instead, the objectives should be small, manageable stuff that you have full power to control. Have you consumed five fruit and veggie servings today? That's one goal achieved. What about 8 hours of sleep; have you got them in? If so, you can cross them off your list.

Gravitate to Positivity

It is vital to surround yourself with the Good. Doing so offers you a relaxing, socially healthy environment to invest in yourself. Don't be afraid to ask for help or support.

Rethink Punishments and Rewards

Remember that making healthier decisions is a way to practice self-care. Food is not a reward, and a workout is not a penalty. They are all necessary to take care of your body and to make you do the best you can. You deserve both.

Taking a few minutes at the start of your exercise or at the beginning of your day to calm down and simply concentrate on breathing will help you set your goals, communicate with your body, and even reduce the stress response of your body.

24 Hour Goals

Having patience is essential when you are losing weight. Plus, if you concentrate on reaching genuinely reachable targets, such as taking 10.000 steps each day, you don't need to be caught up in your list of goals. New accomplishments come in every 24 hours; concentrate on those.

Identify 'Troublesome Thoughts'

Identify the feelings that bring you problems, and seek to prevent and change them. Let them stop intentionally by saying 'no' out loud. It may sound silly, but that simple action breaks your chain of thought and helps you to introduce a new, safer one.

Don't step on the scale

Even though stepping on the scale to check on your progress is not bad, many people often associate it with negative thoughts. If you know the number on the scale will lead to negative and self-destructive thoughts, then you should avoid it, at least until you are in a place where the number on the scale doesn't affect your mental health.

Get to learn how to cope

Many of your problems with weight loss are from your physiological reactions to stress. Most times, you crave spaghetti or candy when you have a bad day. Or you order a pizza because there was nothing to cook for dinner. Or give up on losing weight when work gets busy or when you get to some other stressful season of life.

When you want to lose weight, life doesn't just continue effortlessly without stress. Sadly, life will never be secure, and there will always be pain. Consequently, if you fall off track each time, life does not go your way, then it is time you learn new coping strategies. The goal is to maintain a healthy lifestyle and lose weight, no matter the obstacles life throws our way.

Eliminate the clutter and the chaos

What do clutter and chaos have to do with weight loss? It's tough to picture a happier future when you are surrounded by confusion and noise. Clutter and confusion build hot zones, and when attempting to escape hot zones, it's challenging to develop new patterns and behaviors.

Concentrate on solutions and not explanations

A proactive approach that has been effective in the weight loss process is relying on options instead of excuses. You may be using excuses because you're scared of failing. So you say something like, "I can't get to the gym at that time" or "I 'm sick" or "That exercise never worked for me" instead of falling into an exercise routine. It offers you the freedom to either give up or not try at all. Failure, however, is part of the process. Failure is Good. And instead of making yourself give up, grant yourself the approval to lose. To succeed, you have to be ok with failure, not just at losing weight but in life in general.

Or you are using excuses for being lazy

Another excuse you give is that you are not ready. You say you want to lose weight, but your explanation says something different. You are not prepared to make the necessary changes to your food habits, prioritize sleep, manage your hot zones, and make time to schedule and prepare meals.

Fresh is best

There are certain occasions where fresh or raw food is not an option, but fresh vegetables and fruits are a perfect way to curb your appetite while receiving essential nutrients and avoiding fats. Because fiber is an indigestible but healthy material, technically, it fills you up and keeps hunger away for a long time. Plus, it will help you to manage your glucose levels and cholesterol. Shakes, energy bars, and juices are not as good as fresh foods. They are filled with plenty of proper nutrients and are intended to supply you while still low in calories, but food processing removes many of the antioxidants and fibers from them; that what makes fresh food so powerful. Maybe you still want to stock healthy energy bars on a shelf in the case of a hunger emergency. However, fresh food will always be the first preference.

Only eat plenty

If you're only worried about weight loss, you're not focusing on being healthy. Instead, you're pursuing a picture of what you want to look like, whether it's excellent for you. Develop a commitment to eat well enough. Eating healthy means giving yourself the energy you need to go through the day. It is about developing a lifestyle that will be able to support you long past your golden years. Eating too little doesn't make you fit, even if your waistline does shrink. Just take a look at what you eat all day long and write it down. Keep a diet log. Do you get sufficient calories? Is there a balance between the types of food you eat? This will ensure that you make healthy lifestyle choices instead of a fast, unhealthy fix.

Talk with your doctor

Any improvement in lifestyle should be made with feedback from your doctor. There will be many blogs selling the perfect diet. However, the fact is that our bodies are different, and the needs of everyone are different. Make sure to talk to a professional who is knowledgeable of your medical history to get the best results in your attempt to begin a healthy lifestyle. They can thus help you in making choices that are right for you. Your doctor may recommend a healthy heart diet if you have high cholesterol. Or, they might recommend a higher calorie intake if you are incredibly active in supporting your exercise. Regardless, you should never change your eating habits without consulting your primary care physician first.

How You Can Tell Change Is Happening

Although you should be pursuing a change in lifestyle with the awareness that real-lasting transition takes time, however, you want to see results at some stage. So how can you say the change that you've worked so hard for is happening?

Finally, if your attitude has changed, you shouldn't feel so compelled to overeat. You should eat an adequate amount when you are hungry — just enough to make you feel full. When you feel full, you should stop. You're not supposed to feel pressure to clean your plate, finish the box or have dessert just because it's there. Look back at the first things you wrote in your journal of change when you started this journey. Compare those things today with the way you talk about health and life. Don't be so worried about which notch you use in your belt. Then look at the effect on your health in the long run.

Chapter 2:

What happens to the body of a menopausal woman?

It must be said that a balanced diet has been carried out in life and there are no major weight fluctuations; this will no doubt be a factor that supports women who are going through menopause, but that it is not a sufficient condition to present with classic symptoms that are felt, which can be classified according to the period experienced. In fact, we can distinguish between the pre-menopausal phase, which lasts around 45 to 50 years, and is physiologically compatible with a drastic reduction in the production of the hormone estrogen (responsible for the menstrual cycle, which actually starts irregularly). This period is accompanied by a series of complex and highly subjective endocrine changes. Compare effectively: headache, depression, anxiety, and sleep disorders.

When someone enters actual menopause, estrogen hormone production decreases even more dramatically, the range of the symptoms widens, leading to large amounts of the hormone, for example, to a certain class called catecholamine adrenaline. The result of these changes is a dangerous heat wave, increased sweating, and the presence of tachycardia, which can be more or less severe.

Although menopause causes major changes that greatly change a woman's body and soul, metabolism is one of the worst. In fact, during menopause, the absorption and accumulation of sugars and triglycerides changes, and it is easy to increase some clinical values such as cholesterol and triglycerides, which lead to high blood pressure or arteriosclerosis. In addition, many women often complain of disturbing circulatory disorders and local edema, especially in the stomach. It also makes weight gain easier, even though you haven't changed your eating habits.

The ideal diet for menopause

In cases where disorders related to the arrival of menopause become difficult to manage, drug or natural therapy under medical supervision may be necessary. The contribution given by a correct diet at this time can be considerable; in fact, given the profound variables that come into play, it is necessary to modify our food routine, both in order not to be surprised by all these changes and to adapt in the most natural way possible.

In fact, they are also responsible for the classic hourglass shape of most women, which consists of depositing fat mainly on the hips, which begins to fail with menopause. As a result, we go from a gynoid condition to an android one, with an adipose increase localized on the belly. In addition, the metabolic rate of disposal is reduced; this means that even if you do not change your diet and eat the same quantities of food as you always have, you could experience weight gain, which will be more marked in the presence of bad habits or irregular diet.

The digestion is also slower and intestinal function becomes more complicated. This further contributes to swelling as well as the occurrence of intolerance and digestive disorders which have never been disturbed before. Therefore, the beginning will be more problematic and difficult to manage during this period. The distribution of nutrients must be different: reducing the amount of low carbohydrate, which is always preferred not to be purified, helps avoid the peak of insulin and at the same time maintains stable blood sugar.

These molecules are divided into three main groups, and the foods that contain them should never be missing on our tables: isoflavones, present mainly in legumes such as soy and red clover; lignans, of which flax seeds and oily seeds, in general, are particularly rich; coumestans, found in sunflower seeds, beans, and sprouts. A calcium supplementation will be necessary through cheeses such as parmesan, dairy products such as yogurt, egg yolk, some vegetables such as rocket, Brussels sprouts, broccoli, spinach, asparagus; legumes; dried fruit such as nuts, almonds, or dried grapes.

Excellent additional habits that will help to regain well-being may be: limiting sweets to sporadic occasions, thus drastically reducing sugars (for example, by giving up sugar in coffee and getting used to drinking it bitterly); learn how to dose alcohol a lot (avoiding spirits, liqueurs, and aperitif drinks) and choose only one glass of good wine when you are in company, this because it tends to increase visceral fat which is precisely what is going to settle at the level abdominal. Clearly, even by eating lots of fruit, it is difficult to reach a high carbohydrate quota as in a traditional diet. However, a dietary plan to follow can be useful to have a more precise indication on how to distribute the foods. Obviously, one's diet must be structured in a personal way, based on specific metabolic needs and one's lifestyle.

Understanding of Metabolism and Fasting

Many people think that skipping meals will make your body adapt to save energy by reducing its metabolic rate. It is well known that very long periods without food can cause a drop in metabolism. Moreover, studies have shown that fasting will improve the metabolism for short periods, not slow it down.

Does Intermittent Fasting slow your metabolism?

The definite answer is yes, but no more than other methods of weight loss. Nonetheless, if you can also maintain lean muscle, the effect on metabolism may be negligible. Nonetheless, relatively few studies focused specifically on intermittent fasting and metabolism and no long-term research. There is still a lot of that we don't know as such.

But, even with the limitations of current research, it's clear that there's no need to avoid intermittent fasting due to potential metabolism impacts. Intermittent fasting indeed remains a powerful weight loss option, and many people find it effective. It is also worth noting that the weight-loss process itself can decrease metabolism. This pattern may be a significant reason why many people who have lost a great deal of weight end up.

Your metabolic rate works like in a positive feedback loop—you eat more, you weigh more, you need more energy to keep that weight, your metabolic rate will be higher, and you need to eat more food to maintain the balance again. If you eat fewer calories than your TDEE due to fasting, dieting, or eating less, you will naturally lose some weight. If you repeat this pattern of putting less fuel into your body than its homeostatic set point, it will eventually down-regulate the requirements of the body for that energy that it does not get and become more preservative and more efficient with what it has. This will result in a slightly lower TDEE simply because your body needs less food. Image outcome for metabolism feedback loop Fasting down the metabolism is also mostly the result of actually eating less food or losing body weight, which will eventually decrease the body's caloric intake homeostasis as well.

Funny enough, 48-hour fasting reportedly accelerates the metabolism by 3-14 percent. My theory is that the first days you're still running on your current TDEE when you start a fast, which causes a slight bump in energy expenditure, but after a while, you're going to lower it down as a natural defensive response. Fasting more than seven days will undoubtedly lower your demands on metabolism and protein. That is where your body goes into conservation mode and wants to keep as much energy as possible.

Intermittent fasting can energize your metabolism to burn fat and help you lose weight, which gives your digestive system a rest. The trick is balancing fasting with a healthy diet and exercise and not taking it to extremes. If you have some health concerns, see your doctor before you try a fast one.

Eliminates Wastes

"The Complete Idiot's Fasting Guide" states that one way to improve your metabolism by helping your body eliminate all the waste and toxins that accumulate from healthy eating and drinking is by fasting.

Activates Human Growth Hormone

According to the Lean Look website, periodic 24-hour fasts are particularly beneficial since your body releases growth hormone after one has fasted for about 18 hours, which helps the body to burn fat and retain muscle.

Regulates Digestion

This will affect your ability to metabolize your food and burn fat if your digestion is slow. "Fasting: The Ultimate Diet" states that intermittent fasts can control digestion and promote healthy bowel function, increasing metabolism.

Improves Eating Habits

Daily fasts can change your attitude about food according to "Fasting: The Ultimate Diet." You will gain insight into your diet rather than being reliant on it and decide what your body requires for optimum work. Precise feeding energizes your metabolism.

Slows Aging

Fasting will delay the aging process by giving the body a break from regular digestion, according to "Fasting: The Ultimate Diet." This is important since one of the main effects of aging is a slower metabolism. The younger the body is, the quicker and more effective the fat-burning capacity of your metabolism.

How does Intermittent Fasting Effect Metabolism?

This is a particular type of diet that, for some people at least, is effective for weight loss. An approach is essentially a form of dietary autophagy, and as a result, hunger is the focus. One of the most used types of intermittent fasting, for example, is the 16:8 diet, in which you only eat for 8 hours a day. While it may sound tough, many people find the food surprisingly easy. Yet, one of the questions most debated is: Does intermittent fasting slow metabolism?

Short-Term Fasting and Metabolism

The conventional idea is that you will slow down your metabolism by skipping food or fasting because your body has to make the things that it has to last longer. Cambridge Diet Feedback That is true in the long run. Further, if you dramatically reduce your calorie intake over an extended period or go a long time without food, this pattern makes sense for your metabolism. Metabolism is, after all, a reference to the speed with which the body burns fuel. If your reserves are low, it is not likely to be as fast.

A short-term easy, though, is not the same thing. Indeed, some research has demonstrated that this practice can increase metabolism. One explanation for this may be that short-term fasting activates a norepinephrine hormone that can enhance fat burning. Also, many hormones have been related to short-term fasting.

Insulin is one such example. Having too much insulin can make weight loss much more difficult because insulin tells the body to store fat effectively. Research shows that intermittent fasting can help lower levels of insulin. Another important hormone is the growth hormone of humans, which can aid fat loss. Research suggests that this hormone will increase dramatically during fasting and helps maintain muscle mass as well.

Additionally, it is unlikely that the intermittent fasting approach will have the same impact as a very low-calorie diet. A 16:8 variation of the menu, for example, also means you're going a little longer without food than you would otherwise. Similarly, a variety of 5:2 only has two low-calorie days every week.

The Impacts Depend on Body Composition

Intermittent fasting is a weight-loss process. Further, as a result, it could potentially lead to both the loss of lean muscle and fat. This issue is popular across weight-loss approaches, particularly those that cut calories or protein intake drastically. For safety and metabolism, muscle mass is very significant.

Specifically, having leaner muscle can play a key role in increasing metabolism and is also correlated with longevity. Yes, working to improve lean muscle is a critical piece of advice for improving metabolism. Doing so can involve getting more protein in your diet or working out (primarily through exercises for resistance). Multiple studies have now indicated that intermittent fasting impacts lean body mass similarly to calorie restriction. Furthermore, this means that intermittent fasting can have a negative effect on your body composition but nothing more than a simple limit on calories. Through that process, intermittent fasting may potentially reduce metabolism.

Chapter 3:

Practical Advice to accelerate weight loss with intermittent fasting

It can be tough to follow a diet. It can be even tougher to follow one, which involves fasting. And just the thought of intentionally skipping a meal is enough for some to be hungry, if not worse.

Still, many people are up for the challenge. Then what's the secret of making this work?

And in an environment where several of the trending diets require many numbers, It stands out as being pretty easy to understand. It does not involve calorie counting, macros, or ketone measurement. You can eat a vast majority of what you'd like during a specific time window, while most programs suggest eating healthy when you eat.

Whether you're struggling with a slow metabolism, more sedentary behavior, or you've let your eating habits slip; weight loss can become daunting once you hit 50 years of age.

Combine these variables with injuries or medical problems, and it may seem difficult to hit the gym to preserve your waistline. Moreover, research shows that weight loss after 50 is still possible due, among other smart choices, to healthy habits and regular exercise.

Eat out less

"We're at a higher risk of weight gain as we age because of our declining metabolism and increasing hormones," says Kirsten David, an EduPlated dietitian. There are certain foods at all costs which you should stop. This one contributes 150 percent to your blood sugar.

"And there are many mental and social obstacles above [age] 50 that can also keep us from losing weight. Further, Start making healthy changes now and form new healthy habits to avoid weight gain from occurring. "David says many people over the age of 50 go out to eat more often because there is less need to prepare because of the children being grown and out of the house.

Make sure that you get enough sleep

"Sleep is necessary for a healthy weight because two hormones, leptin, and ghrelin, are released during sleep and play a significant role in controlling appetite. Sleeplessness perturbs the cycle and induces metabolic instability in which the body confuses exhaustion hunger— not a good thing! My prescription is to sleep for seven to eight hours and take a low dose of melatonin if needed for relief. Moreover, let go of old "rules" about weight loss and cultivate a mindset of wellness.

"But that doesn't mean mission impossible to lose weight over age 50 years. Diet and exercise are essential, but the common mistake I see is that people eat and work out in the same manner, they did when they were younger and wonder why they don't see results. Those who are over 50 can't eat and exercise the same way they did when they were 30.

"Build a spa mentality," Vercelletto advises. "Being over [age] 50 isn't a death sentence— in reality, many of us now have more time to look after ourselves. It's all super important to have a healthy weight, eat properly, not smoke, and reduce alcohol consumption.

When you get enough sleep, you become healthier, and your overall well-being is guaranteed.

When we sleep, the body operates certain functions in the body that helps burn calories and improves the metabolic rate.

Start Small

For beginners, you can start by having your food at 8 pm, for example, and having nothing again until 8 am the next day. It will be easier since sleep is incorporated into your eating window.

Avoid Stress

Intermittent might be hard to do if you are stressed. This is because stress can trigger an overindulgence of food in some people. It is also easier to feed on junk when stressed to feel better. That's why when on intermittent fasting, you are advised to avoid if not control your stress levels.

Keep Off Flavored Drinks

Most flavored drink says that they are low in sugar, but in the real sense, they are not. Flavored drinks contain artificial sweeteners, which will affect your health negatively. They will also increase your appetite, causing you to overeat, and this will make you gain weight instead of losing.

Increased Healthy Fats

Since the intermittent diet increases ketones in your body, you want to increase healthy fats in your diet. Ketones are responsible for supporting your body in using fat as a fuel instead of sugars. This means that you need to have a healthy amount of fats for the ketones to work on your body effectively. This might seem counterintuitive since you want to burn fats, but it is actually essential.

It is important that you choose healthy fats for this, as this will keep your fuel clean and effective. Filling up on unhealthy fats can be dangerous as it can actually have a negative impact on heart and blood health.

This is why I chose a simple keto meal plan for you.

Avoiding Sugary and Starchy Foods

If you are going to eat something sweet, however, opt for fruits over processed sugars. This will ensure that you are maintaining healthy blood sugar levels. This will also help your body continue using ketones and fat as fuel instead of sugar and carbs.

Healthy meals should be your focus. They will help you get the required nutrients like vitamins, which will give you more energy during the fasting period.

When you hear your stomach growl, it may sound like there's no chance you'll be alive or be able to go through any more hours without eating. Tune in with the hunger warning. Ask yourself if the hunger is just because you are bored or a pang of actual hunger. If it's just boredom, then get something to distract you.

If you are really hungry but do not feel weak or light-headed, drink a warm mint tea, since peppermint is recognized to lower cravings, or take water to help hold your stomach until your eating window.

If you've been doing this for quite a while and your hunger pangs are still more intense than ever during your fasting windows, you may need to do some thinking. You need to either incorporate more nutrient- or calorie-dense items during your eight-hour eating window or realize that intermittent fasting might not be the best plan for you.

Eat when necessary

Theoretically, extreme hunger and tiredness ought not to happen if you follow the 16:8 fasting strategy (maybe the most common one). But if you're feeling extremely light-headed, then your body might be trying to tell you something. You are probably hypoglycemic, and you need to get something in your stomach — and this is ok. By description, fasting means removing some food, so you shouldn't get yourself worked up for breaking your fast with a little bite. Opt for a protein-rich snack like a few pieces of chicken thighs or one or two hard-boiled eggs.

Stay hydrated

Even if you're fasting, taking bevies like coffee, tea, and drinking water (without milk) is not only permitted but also urged.

You can set reminders during the day and especially during your fasting windows to drink lots of liquids. Strive to take at least 2 or 3 liters per day.

Staying hydrated when you're fasting is a must. It will not only protect you from being dehydrated; it will prevent constipation and help you in dealing with hunger. Staying hydrated is essential because your oral intake is less than it was, and your body needs lots of fluid to work efficiently.

You don't have to take only plain water. You can also make calorie-free herbal teas such as chamomile or peppermint that can help you stay hydrated while maintaining your fast

Break your fast slowly and steadily

Since you are staying many hours without food, you may start feeling like a vacuum eager to suck everything on your plate. When eating, you must chew adequately and eat gradually to allow the digestive system to absorb the food entirely.

Avoid overeating

Just because you are in your eating window doesn't mean you should eat everything in sight. Overeating doesn't only cause you to become uncomfortable and bloated, but it can also thwart the weight-loss plans. It's not merely the amount of food on your plate that can keep you full for long; instead, it's what's on your plate.

Keep the meals balanced

Having a balanced combination of protein, carbohydrates, good fats will eventually help you lose weight and stay clear of intense hunger while fasting.

Go for fruits with a low-glycemic index that is ingested, digested, and absorbed by the body more gradually, creating a lower and slower increase of blood glucose.

Look for a healthy meal that's easy to digest and not one packed with candy or simple carbs that will raise your blood sugar.

Strategically use Caffeine

Caffeine can reduce hunger pangs and your urge to eat for a short time." You could use this to your benefit while fasting by beginning daily with a small glass of black coffee. This will not break your fast but can keep you feeling less hungry and energized. Don't overdo it, as it could lead to headaches, muscle tremors, and irritability.

Play around with different eating times

You have to look at different fasting methods to see which one is suitable for you. For instance, if your day starts early, you could eat soon, like at 10 am a.m. to 6 pm, and fast from then to 10 am the next day.

Another option is to ease yourself gradually by eating breakfast later every day to increase your fasting strength.

Steer clear of fasts lasting for 24 hours

It is not advisable to do a full day fast as it can lead to higher fatigue, appetite, and food intake — and, therefore, weight gain.

If you aim to lose weight, then evaluating your total caloric consumption and focusing on slowing it down might be more effective than fasting for an extended period (especially if you're the sort to binge after). There are no more advantages to fasting for 24 hours than everyday caloric restriction.

Adapt your workout routine

You should probably work out if you're following a fasting diet. However, you ought to be conscious of what sorts of activity you're doing and when. If you want to exercise in your fasting window, consider doing it early in the morning since you have the most strength then.

Keep track of your journey

Believe it or not, maintaining a food journal may aid you in managing your fasting diet. While you may not document as many meals as you consume, you may regularly track information such as any thoughts and signs (hunger, fatigue, etc.) that occur while you're fasting. It will help you gauge your success.

Chapter 4:

Intermittent Fasting – One of the Best Ways to Cut Fat

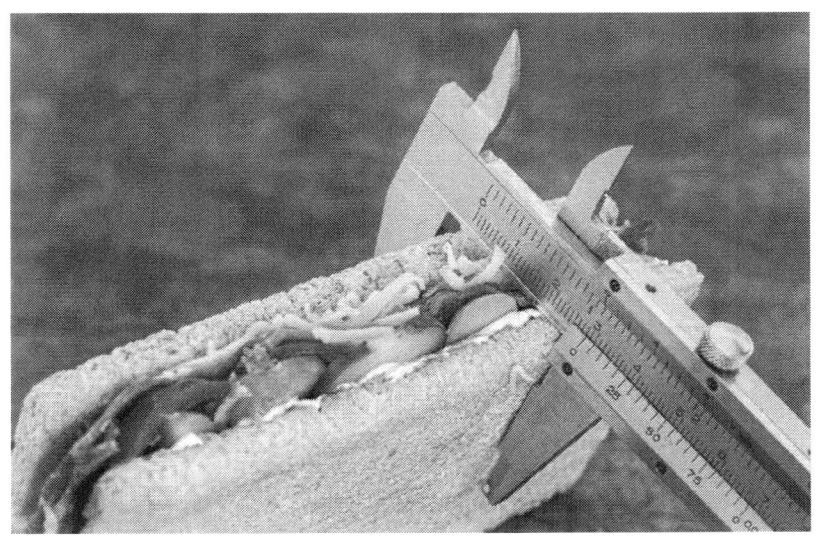

"The Best And The Fastest Way To Lose Weight"

This is a catch phrase you might have heard in the commercials of most weight loss programs and hence hearing it once again may not create any spark in your mind. However, it is one of the most sought-after catchphrases among people battling obesity. This phrase shows a ray of hope to all the people facing the brunt of obesity. At least they see another way to try to shed the menace of excess weight.

The problem is that most of the weight loss programs are designed at best only to try to keep you tied in your current weight category and believe me, even that is not a mean task. Our current lifestyle has become such that even maintaining the current weight is not an easy task for an already obese person.

An overweight person may have some option to lose weight but an already obese person has very few of them. For an obese person, the current weight in itself acts as a counter force. It limits all kind of physical activities that can help in losing weight. Obesity also brings with itself a number of health issues like diabetes, hypertension, cardiovascular diseases, etc. that again reduce the ability to engage in any kind of strenuous activity.

Hence, the options with obese people are far and few between. Therefore, they fall prey to such advertisements and eventually face disappointment.

Intermittent Fasting

Intermittent Fasting is a real ray of hope for such people. It is the blast of light at the end of the dark tunnel.

The first and the most important thing to understand is that intermittent fasting isn't a commercial product. It is free of cost and you are the sole party involved with the process. Hence, there is no one else to blame.

It is a natural process of mechanism that helps in losing weight and cutting the visceral fat in your body. If you are suffering from obesity, it can transform your life completely.

It is no magic concept. It is a scientific process of burning the body fat naturally. Hence, it requires discipline and determination. You will have to become conscious of your eating choices and lifestyle habits. However, the results would be outstanding and hence you would more than you asked for in return for your efforts.

One important thing that you must remember is that it is a natural process and hence the results would take their own time. There would be no chemical or steroid induced results and hence you may take a bit longer than usual to experience the change but it would surely be there.

Why Intermittent Fasting Works while Others Fail?

The biggest problem with most weight loss measure is that they treat weight gain to be a too simplistic process. People believe that by simply reducing the calorie intake they can force the body to burn the stored fat in the body. It doesn't work that way.

Diets

For instance, let us assume that your body spends 2000 calories a day even if you sit idle at your home.

This energy is spent in breathing, remaining awake, carrying out other life processes, etc.

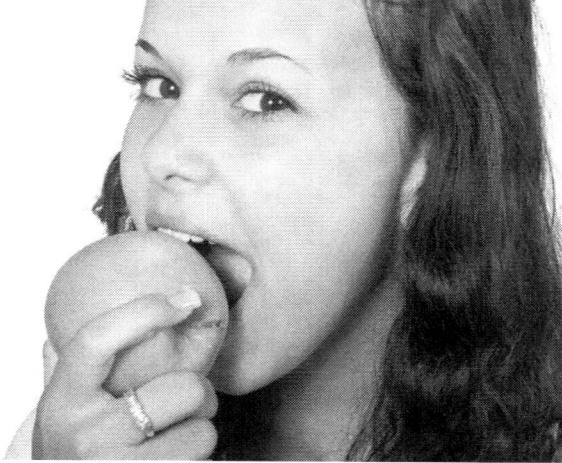

Now, if you start consuming only 1500 calories a day, that would create a shortage of 500 calories. No doubt it would be tough in the beginning but you can do at least this much for a leaner body.

However, even if you pass through this ordeal, you'd find no significant change in your weight or fat. Although you would feel more sluggish, lethargic, and irritable. All this would happen because your body sensed the shortage of energy and lowered its energy needs

Your metabolic functions get slow and your body starts conserving energy even more aggressively as it senses an oncoming famine like situation. It is the survival mechanism. The body has learned this trick through the evolutionary process spanning millions of years.

It is a fail-safe mechanism put in place by the mother nature to ensure better survival chances. However, this very mechanism can make losing weight through diets a miserable idea.

When you start dieting, you may witness drastic weight loss in the beginning stage. This happens because your body dumps a lot of water. The water in the body besides other functions also plays an important role in regulating body temperature. But, it also uses up a lot of energy too.

When your body feels a shortage of energy supply, the first thing it does is that it dumps the excess water. The priority of your body is no longer to keep you warm and comfortable. Its main concern becomes ensuring survival through the rough patch.

However, this loss of water weight is temporary. As soon as you would resume normal diet or start taking normal calories the water weight would come back. Such loss of weight isn't effective or helpful in any way at all.

Therefore, diets fail miserably in bringing any significant result.

Diet is only a way to send a signal to your body that there is a scarcity of energy and the shortage can be indefinite and hence the body can go in overdrive to conserve energy. It would stop spending any excess energy.

Exercise

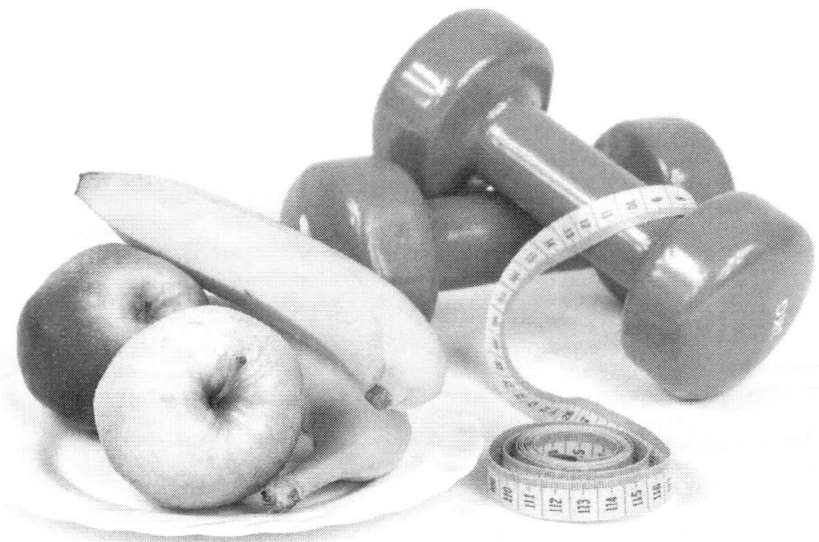

Exercise is a great way to burn calories. It helps you in burning the excess fat from specific areas. However, there is a significant problem with obese or morbidly obese people that they may not find the inclination or stamina to undertake the amount of exercise in the beginning. Even slightly overweight people find the exercise routine tough to adjust in their daily schedule.

Exercise requires great grit and determination. One needs to have that right frame of mind to ensure fast weight loss through exercise. This is generally not the case with most people and hence they find this route difficult.

Medication

It is not uncommon for people to look for medical help to counter their weight. Medical science has made groundbreaking progress in the past century and it has the power to cure most problems. However, obesity is not one among them. Obesity is a lifestyle disorder and hence simply taking pills cannot solve the issue. Some people also fall prey to poorly researched products boasting about the results but they end up losing their hard- earned money and confidence. There is no magic way to lose weight. It is a lifestyle disorder and the solution would only come when you commit to a lifestyle change and start practicing it.

Surgery

Bariatric surgeries have emerged as the new fad in the weight loss segment. The people suffering from morbid obesity may have a ray of hope there. There are several bariatric procedures like gastric banding and gastric sleeve that offer some relief but experience has shown that the results don't last very long if they are not followed up by lifestyle changes. These procedures only provide temporary relief by reducing your food and nutrition absorption abilities. The body adjusts itself to the restriction pretty fast and if you don't make serious lifestyle changes weight would come back much faster. These surgeries are very costly and can only be performed on selected patients suffering from morbid obesity. They are not as simple as cosmetic procedures. Several factors including your overall health would have to be considered by the doctor before carrying out the procedure. These surgeries create a lot of limitations and also carry many risks as in case of other surgical procedure.

Intermittent Fasting - The Saviour

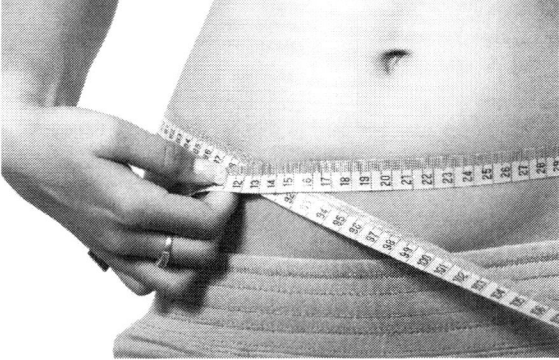

Intermittent fasting has gained great popularity in a very short period of time. The only reason behind this popularity is its ability to deliver results through simple measures.
Intermittent fasting is such a simple concept that you don't need to do anything special to make it a part of your life. It isn't a concept of adding anything to your life but removing a few excess things from it.
It has two basic elements at the core 1. fasting and 2. doing it intermittently. Fasting as we know is the state of depriving yourself of food. It is as simple as that. Intermittent means that you're eating and fasting periods would be sporadic. You will have shorter eating periods in a day and longer fasting periods. Simply by creating the gap in your eating and fasting schedule, you can bring about a sea change in your health.

Intermittent fasting can help in bringing down insulin resistance, high blood pressure and risk of several diseases by influencing your system in a positive way. Your gut would able to function better and your food intake gets controlled. Your overall health biomarkers would show considerable improvements. All these results can be achieved by simply bringing changes in your eating and fasting patterns. This is a phenomenon that has caught the attention of people trying to lose weight and the whole world is watching it with awe and excitement.

The world has started acknowledging the benefits intermittent fasting has to offer. There has been some serious research on the topic and the results are very promising.

Fasting as a religious concept has also been present in society for very long. It has been practiced in almost all religions across the globe. For instance, the Muslims follow short fasts for a whole month during Ramadan. Studies have shown that practicing these fasts leads to significant improvement in blood sugar levels, hypertension, cardiovascular health, and insulin sensitivity.

Buddhist monks practice rigorous fasting. They are known to live a healthier and fulfilling life. The Jains in India follow a lifestyle that's a form of intermittent fasting. It has helped them remain fit and healthy despite their pretty sedentary lifestyle for centuries.

These are simply some prominent examples where intermittent fasting is followed as a form of religious practice. It has got ingrained into the lifestyle and is helping the followers in a great way.

The best thing about intermittent fasting is that it is very easy to follow. It isn't limiting and doesn't make you feel trapped inside a cage like one feels when following diets.

Although it isn't fair to draw parallels between two practices as everything has positives and negatives. Yet, diets have ruled the wellness industry for a very long period. They mesmerized the weight loss enthusiasts and people followed diets in droves.

Some people got results very fast while others completely failed to get any kind of result. However, one thing was common to all and that was desperation to get off diets. The diets always had a time limit and people waited impatiently for the diets to end. They saw the freedom to eat at the end what they had been missing all the while. They felt starved, frustrated, and highly irritable. Therefore, as soon as they got off the diet most people did binge eating.

Studies show that more than 80% of people who followed a diet of any kind either regained their actual weight or gained even more. Failure of such a rate should be considered catastrophic for any process and yet people follow diets.

They are constricting in nature and create temptation that acts as a counter force. You are always thinking about the things that you can't eat as you have been denied permission to eat them. This is how the basic human psyche works.

Intermittent fasting is relaxed. It imposes restrictions of time on you as your eating hours are limited. However, it puts no specific restriction of the kinds of things you can eat.

Intermittent fasting focuses more on when to eat rather than what to eat.

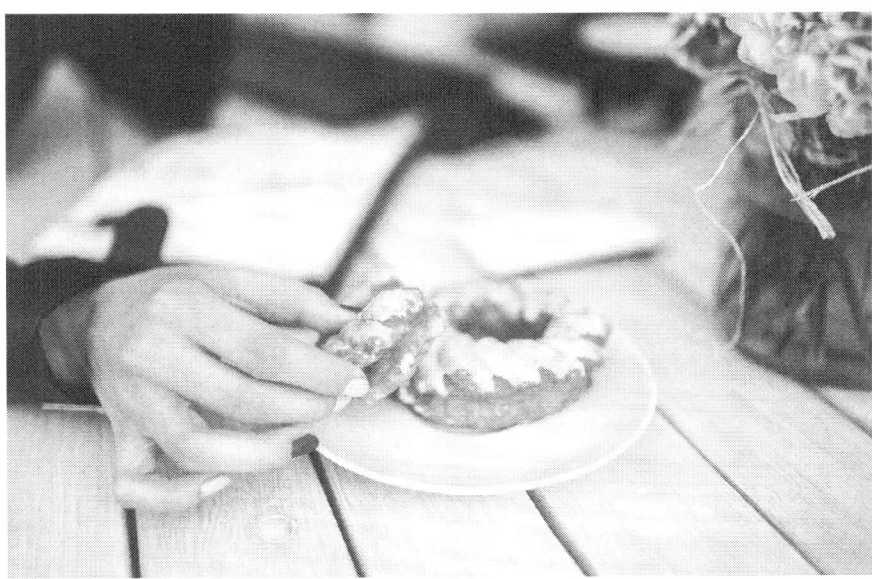

Therefore, it eliminates the possibility of temptation and resultant binge eating. Intermittent fasting starts a powerful process of fat burning that will not only help you in getting slimmer and leaner but will also help you in getting healthier. It is a holistic way to achieve better health without compromising on anything.

Before we begin to understand the ways in which intermittent fasting helps you in losing weight and cutting the fat, it is important to understand the reasons leading to obesity. This understanding will help you in not only losing the weight easily but also in keeping it off permanently.

Chapter 5:

Poor Eating Habits - Cause of Debacle

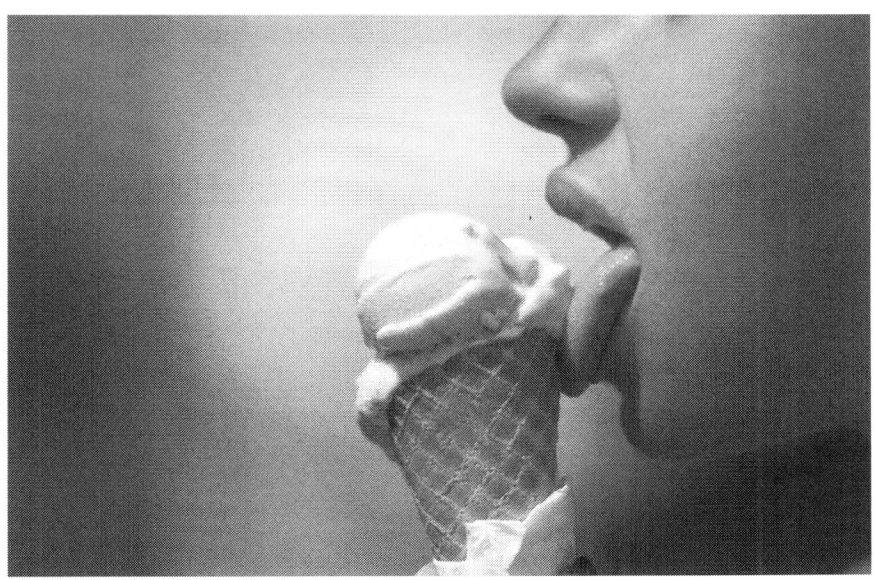

Food is a very important part of our lives. Getting food to the table has been a constant endeavor of the human race. Getting some sort of food security has been the grand goal of human progress. It is the only thing for which humankind kept evolving continuously from hunter-gatherer to cultivator and then to processor and manufacturer. We have come a long way in this direction.

Today, a greater part of the world is free from food scarcity. We don't have to gather our tools and go on a hunt every day to find food. We can simply order it and have months supply stacked at our homes without much effort.

However, this comfort has also brought some serious problems too. The abundance of food has also changed our eating patterns. Unregulated access to food means that we can eat anytime we want. This is something that hasn't been a part of our lives for long and it is causing a lot of problems in our system.

Historical Eating Patterns

Historically, our eating pattern was very simple. Our ancestors were hunter-gatherers. They went out every day to get food. By the end of the day, whatever they could get was distributed among all and comprised the single biggest meal of the day. There were no storage and refrigeration facilities back then and hence whatever food was available was consumed in the single meal.

It meant that people ate in excess amounts and then remained in the fasting state till the next meal that might be available the next day or thereafter. This was the simplest eating pattern with long and forced fasting period and big feast in the end.

Slowly our ancestors found a more reliable way to get food and they started cultivation. It was a tiresome job but gave a higher probability of getting a consistent supply of food. However, it required a lot of hard work and limited food. Till this time, obesity was not the concern of the society.

People died in large numbers all around the globe even due to small issues like fever, infections and insect bites. But, people didn't die of obesity and other lifestyle disorders. Obesity is a fairly new phenomenon that has become so prevalent in this age and time. The main reason behind it is the abundance of food and the careless nature in which we consume it.

The Relation between Random Food Consumption and Health Issues

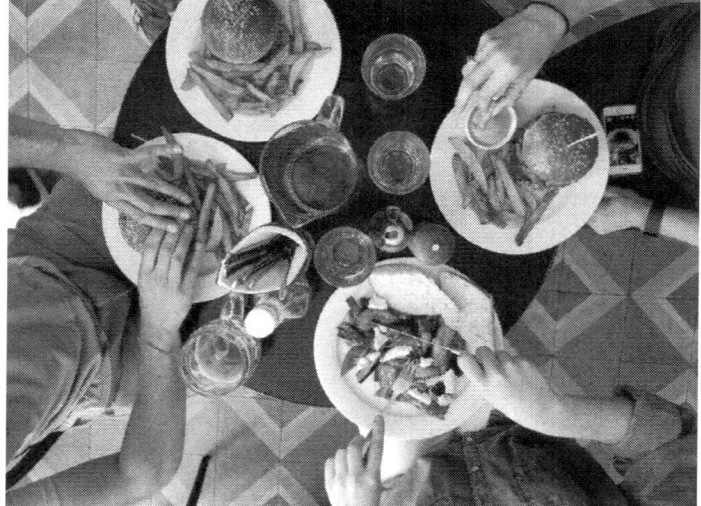

Food provides us life energy. It has a very vital role to play in our body. Therefore, the food we consume needs to be absorbed by our body completely. Our body is like an efficient machine that utilizes most of the food we eat and makes it a part of itself. Only the waste material is secreted out of the body. However, this process is time-consuming and shouldn't be rushed. This is the point where we are making a mistake.

We have got into a habit where we eat things not because we are feeling hungry but because they are available in front of us. Most of the times we eat street food simply because someone is selling it and it looks tempting. The same goes for 6-8 meals a day we consume. All this is without counting the number of times we engage our system by ingesting calories in the form of sweetened beverages, candies, cookies, chips, and other munchies. All these things not only a great number of unwanted calories to your system but also keep your digestive system engaged most of the time.

Almost all forms of medical streams including the conventional and alternative medical streams believe that our digestive system is one of the most crucial systems. Most of the diseases in the body can be avoided if the digestive system keeps working perfectly. It performs some of the most crucial functions and keeps our body healthy and nourished. However, when we start eating after every few hours and keep the digestive system engaged, it is very natural for it to get slow and inefficient. It is the beginning of most of the health issues.

Frequent consumption of meals puts a lot of undue stress on your digestive tract. It affects the functioning of your intestine. Not only this, but the consumption of food at regular intervals also leads to some of the major health issues like insulin resistance. It is a disorder that may not be known as a disease in itself but is behind several major disorders like diabetes, hypertension, heart diseases, liver malfunction, and stress. It is also a major reason behind fast weight gain. Simply by reducing insulin resistance, one can ensure freedom from a large number of health issues. Intermittent fasting is one of the best ways to reverse insulin resistance and bring insulin sensitivity that could help you in leading a healthy life.

Eating food at regular intervals is neither good for your gut nor for your weight loss measures. By practicing intermittent fasting you can easily ensure both the things. Intermittent fasting is the process of bringing a reasonable gap between your meals. It is a cycle of eating and fasting windows within a day. It is very simple to practice and costs nothing at all.

Chapter 6:

How Intermittent Fasting Works

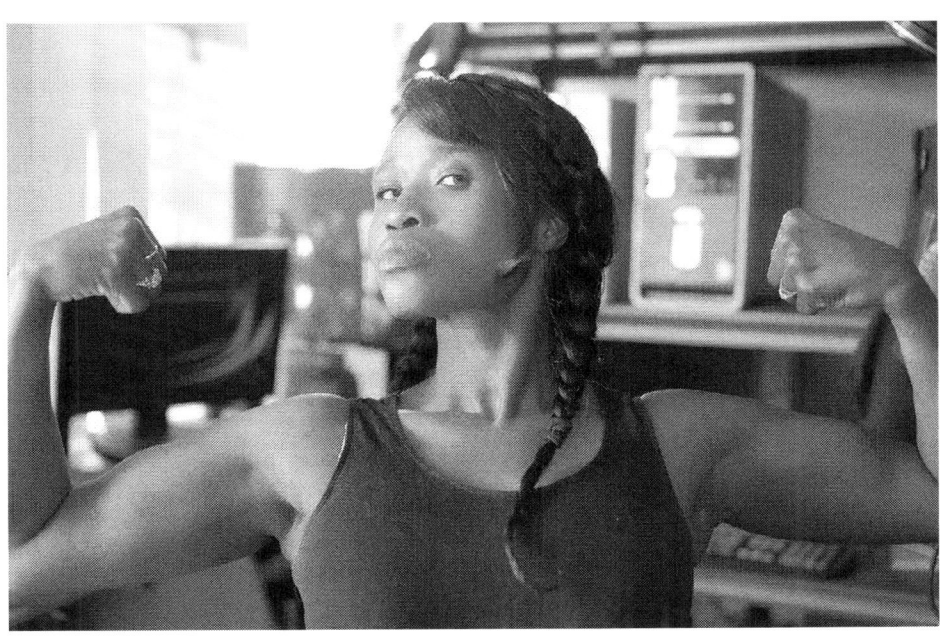

Intermittent Fasting takes off the unwanted load from your internal system. It helps your body in regrouping its strength. Your vital organs get a chance to become more sensitive to responses. All this can happen by simply practicing extended fasting periods in your daily routine.

Excess of things is a major cause of problems in the body. We are keeping our bodies under the constant pressure of work. Eating and drinking may look like a fulfilling exercise but it is a task for the body to process it.
This task keeps the body engaged and doesn't allow it the time to relax. This leads to fatigue and various body functions start developing a kind of resistance.

To understand it in simple words you can take the analogy of cooking something in your kitchen. Let us suppose you have started boiling pasta. Pasta boils in a definite period of time. Neither overcooked pasta is good for eating nor the uncooked one. Now suppose you start cooking pasta and add some more to the same water after 2 minutes. You wait for

2 minutes and add some more. You keep adding more and more pasta after an interval of 2 minutes. In the end, you would be having a mess at your hand. Some of the pasta that was added in the beginning would get overcooked. Some of it would get cooked fairly while most of it would remain undercooked. You would have an unedible pasta in your plate although you boiled it for the desired period and followed the process thoroughly.

We are doing exactly the same with our body. Any specific meal, howsoever insignificant in quantity and light in nature takes a few hours to get digested properly. Experts believe that food takes at least 6-8 hours to pass through our stomach and the small intestine. From here the process gets very slow and the food gets absorbed very slowly. So our body needs longer gaps between meals to process the food properly and absorb all the nutrients. However, we are not giving this time to our body and it is also causing most of the problems.

When we start our day in the morning we start by breakfast or an early morning snack this happens between 7-9 am. Between 11-12 people again have snacks and tea. This is a meal right before lunch which takes place between 1-3 pm. The lunch causes lethargy in most people and hence tea and beverages come to the rescue. The evening snacks between 5-6 pm are also preferred by many people as this allows them late dinner and helps in eliminating hunger. The last meal of the day takes place ideally between 9-11 pm right before bedtime.

This whole routine doesn't give your body any time to relax. Your digestive system is always at work. It never gets those 6-8 hours to completely process a meal before the next one comes. You are simply adding more and more pasta to the same pot and spoiling the whole meal.

The food in our gut is not getting processed properly as our gut holds food items at various stages of processing that get the same treatment. This causes most of the digestive issues. Your body fails to absorb the required nutrients and you have to other option than to take nutrient supplements.
Your insulin levels always remain very high as frequent meals keep spiking blood glucose levels.

Your hunger and satiety hormones start responding in a wacky manner as the differentiation gets difficult.

You get prone to diabetes and insulin resistance in your body increases with time.
It also leads to an increase in your blood pressure and insulin resistance trips other vital parameters.

From chronic inflammation to the overactive release of stress hormones, the body is in a continuous struggle.

All this can happen simply because you choose to eat whenever you liked.

Now, think that you have been doing that for your whole life. Until the body is in teenage, it has a very powerful digestive mechanism and there is a constant release of growth hormones. There is high energy need and hence this doesn't affect us much and there is no significant weight gain. But, once you cross teenage and start leading a bit sedentary life obesity starts kicking in. The digestive process starts getting weak and all the metabolic functions come under great strain.

The first thing intermittent fasting does is that it strengthens your digestive process by reducing the pressure from it. It gives your crucial functions like insulin formation the desired break and your system is able to relax. It is also the system that affects your fat storage and hence your fat burning begins.

Intermittent fasting has a profound impact on most of your body functions and helps them in functioning better.

The next few chapters will explain the ways in which intermittent fasting helps your crucial body functions and how that affects your weight loss and fat burning

Chapter 7:

Lowers Insulin Resistance

What is Insulin?

Insulin is one of the most important hormones in our body. It performs a very crucial function and that is to facilitate absorption of energy by cells. Let us understand this is a simpler way.

Whenever you eat anything, that food gets processed and energy is released in the form of glucose. This glucose is released in the bloodstream and increases your blood sugar levels. Glucose is the simplest form of energy and all the cells in our body can use it directly for producing energy. This means that as soon as you eat or drink anything that contains calories your blood sugar levels rise.

However, there is a catch. Although your cells can use glucose directly for producing the energy they can't absorb it without outside help. You can consider the energy receptors to be locked which need a key for glucose to pass into the cells. Insulin is that key that can help in the process.

Our pancreas releases the insulin hormone as soon as it senses high blood sugar levels to stabilize the blood sugar level at the earliest. This insulin can bind itself with the cells and help in the absorption of energy.

The high blood sugar level is dangerous as it can lead to several health complications and persistent high blood sugar levels can also lead to multiple organ failure. If the blood sugar level remains high in general then it can also thicken the vessels in your vital organs and deteriorate their functioning. This is a reason people suffering from diabetes generally also have other issues like hypertension, heart problems, liver and kidney issues, chronic inflammation, etc.

What is Insulin Resistance?

Insulin resistance is a phenomenon in which the cells stop responding to insulin actively. It means that in spite of high blood sugar levels and ample amount of insulin in the blood, the cells in your body don't open up to receive glucose. This may sound absurd but it happens more often than you can think of.

Suppose there are your grandparents who bring candies for you whenever they come. You'd be super excited whenever they'd come to your home. However, what if they start living next door to you and come to your home several times a day. You may love them all the same but wouldn't be as excited as in the earlier case as it would become a regular affair. Now add to this the fact that they are also keeping an eye at you all the time. You may even start feeling annoyed by their presence and may not show that same speed in opening the door as earlier. If they start interfering in your personal matter or start controlling or keep shouting at you, you may not feel inclined at all to open the door.

The same happens in your body when you are having frequent meals or consuming food or beverages containing calories. As soon as you eat anything it gets processed as glucose and raises your blood sugar level.

Your pancreas releases the insulin hormone to bring down the blood sugar level. But, if you start consuming food or calorific beverages too often your blood sugar level would remain high consistently. This means that the insulin would be knocking the doors of the cells all the time. These cells, in that case, become less sensitive or resistant to the insulin signals.

This creates several problems:

1.   Your blood sugar levels remain high for unreasonably long periods of time. This is dangerous on many levels.

2.   Your pancreas would keep pumping more and more insulin into your blood to lower the blood sugar level.

3.   The insulin levels in your blood that was already high would keep getting higher leading to greater insulin resistance.

Insulin resistance is a very dangerous condition as it leads to several health complications. The longer the blood sugar levels remain higher the greater is the risk of health complications.

The problem is that there is no outside mechanism to solve this problem. With the passage of time, this problem keeps on intensifying.

If your cells are not responding to the insulin signals readily then you would feel energy deprived more often. You'd also feel more lethargic as your blood sugar levels would be higher.

For your body to function optimally it should have insulin sensitivity and not insulin resistance.

Main Cause of Insulin Resistance

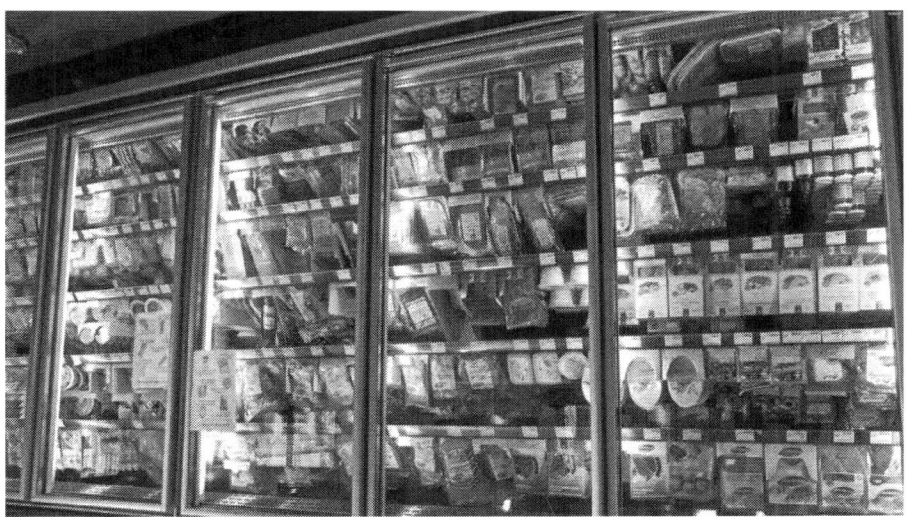

Bad eating habit is the main cause of increasing insulin resistance these days. There was a time when people ate when they felt hungry. Those days are long gone. Now, we eat to celebrate. We eat when we are feeling depressed. We also eat when we are getting bored. We eat to increase the fun of the movies. We eat when we see something tempting being served on the streets. Eating has become yet another important function and then we wonder why we are getting bulkier. Bad eating habits are the chief cause of increasing insulin resistance and also a cause of the rapid rise of obesity in society.

We keep adding calories to our system at very short intervals and keep it overloaded. We also keep the gut engaged all the time. Our pancreas remains overworked as it has to keep pumping insulin all time to counter perennially high levels of blood sugar. Frequent eating is at the root of the problem.

How Does Intermittent Fasting Help in Developing Insulin Sensitivity?

Intermittent fasting is a very simple yet highly effective way to bring normalcy to your system. It helps in reversing insulin resistance and promotes the development of insulin sensitivity.

The root cause of insulin resistance is an overload on the system. The higher the number of meals you consume in a day, the lower is the time your system gets to process those meals. The blood sugar spikes are frequent and that also leads to insulin resistance. Your body slowly and gradually surrenders to the assault and stops reacting proactively to the signals.

Intermittent fasting helps in dealing with the issues that cause insulin resistance. It is a simple process of having shorter eating windows and longer fasting windows. What this means is that your body gets more time to process the meals. The frequent blood sugar spikes also get lower and hence the pancreas can relax a bit.

Your body needs at least 5-8 hours for a single meal to digest. This means that your blood sugar levels would be the highest immediately after consuming the meal and the lowest after 5-8 hours after your last meal. When you start practicing intermittent fasting you will have much shorter eating windows.

For instance, you follow an intermittent fasting protocol where you have an eating window of 8 hours and fasting window of 16 hours. This means that you can have 2-3 meals during the 8 hours eating window but you will have to remain in the fasted state for the rest of the day or night.

This 16-hour fasting window will allow your gut the requisite time to process all the meals properly. Your blood sugar levels would also not see any sudden spike in the fasting window as there will be no calorie intake. This means the pancreas will not have the added responsibility of continuously pumping insulin. The insulin levels are the highest immediately after you have any kind of calorie intake. It takes around 8-12 hours for the insulin levels to go down. This means if you are following a 16-hour fasting window, there will be a significant amount of time when the insulin levels in your body would be the lowest. This single phenomenon helps tremendously in bringing down insulin resistance and developing insulin sensitivity.

When the insulin levels are constantly high in your blood due to frequent intake of food, the cells start reacting to insulin signals poorly. It is like someone is constantly banging at the door and you stop paying attention to it. However, when there are periods when the insulin levels are very low and other periods when the levels are high, the cells start reacting to the insulin signals better.

Intermittent fasting is one of the most important steps towards developing insulin sensitivity.

Getting rid of insulin resistance is very important. It is responsible for most of the problems in your body. It acts as a slow poison for most of the systems and brings you down.

It also plays a very important role in adding to your weight and fat stores. In the next chapter, we will understand the ways in which insulin is responsible for weight gain and high- fat deposits in the body.

Chapter 8:

Lowering Belly Fat and the Role of Insulin

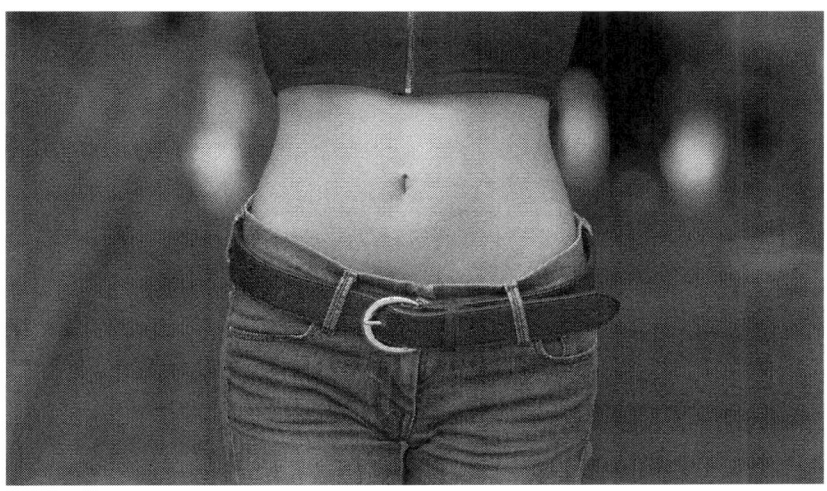

The word insulin points only towards the direction of diabetes in general. Only the people suffering from diabetes feel a direct connection with the name as they need to take insulin shots on a regular basis to control their sugar.

People seldom realize that this hormone may have a direct connection with their weight and fat. If you are gaining a lot of fat around your belly, thighs or on your hips, then insulin is the hormone to blame for it.

Insulin is the main fat storage hormone in your body. It is the hormone that regulates any kind of fat storage in your body. Your body would never shed a gram of fat as long as there is high insulin presence in your body.

Let us first understand the mechanism of fat storage in the body.

- As soon as you consume calories in any form they are converted into glucose.

- This glucose mixes with the blood and raises your blood sugar level.

- Immediately the pancreas senses the high blood sugar levels and pumps insulin in the bloodstream to stabilize the blood sugar levels.

- The job of insulin is to ensure that the blood sugar is not floating around and gets used or stored.

- The primary objective of the insulin hormone is to facilitate maximum absorption of glucose in the cells.

- It signals the cells and binds with them to ensure optimum absorption of glucose.
- Cells can absorb only a limited amount of glucose. They do not have a high storage capacity.
- Insulin then tries to store the remaining glucose in muscles and the liver as glycogen.
- Glycogen is another easy form of energy that your body can use in times of need.
- However, the muscles and liver cannot store a large amount of glycogen.
- In the third stage, the insulin signals the fat cells to store all the remaining blood sugar as fat.

Any amount of fat getting stored in your body is a work of insulin. It is the hormone that regulates all kinds of fat storage. So, if you want to blame your belly tires, insulin is the hormone to take the blame. The main reason behind the failure of most weight loss programs is that they fail to understand this crucial point. As long as there is a high presence of insulin in the body, there will be no fat burning at all. Fat burning and fat storage are two diagonally opposite processes. If you think that you will be able to burn the belly fat after doing a few dozen push-ups while you keep sipping the high-calorie energy drink in the gym, you are wrong. As soon as there is an intake of calories, it will spike your blood sugar level and lead to high insulin levels. The insulin in the body would put all its weight behind storing the excess energy consumed in the form of fat. Hence, there will not be any kind of fat burning. The only way to burn the body fat is to cut-off readily available energy supply and to force the body to go for the stored energy.

How is Intermittent Fasting Different from Dieting?
Although dieting and intermittent fasting may look similar concepts, they are completely different.

Dieting

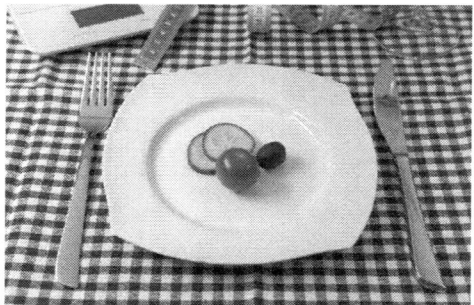

Some Important Facts about Dieting:
- Dieting lowers your calorie intake but it doesn't put any restraints on the number of meals. In fact, most diets support small but frequent meals.

- Diets put too much stress on what to eat and what not to eat. They are not much concerned about the number of times you can eat as long as you remain in the calorie limit.

- By limiting the calories, diets also limit the intake of several important nutrients. This weakens your body and its ability to function optimally goes down.

- Dieting works on the principle that if there is a shortage of energy supply and the energy use is high, the body would start burning the body fat. This idea has several problems.

First, as soon as you limit your energy consumption, your body starts preparing a counter strategy and lowers the energy expenditure. You will need to work extra hard to beat your body in this race. This would make you feel tired, exhausted, and irritated.Second, the science of fat burning is not that simple. As long as there is high insulin presence, your body would remain in fat storage mode and wouldn't transition into the fat burning mode.

Intermittent Fasting

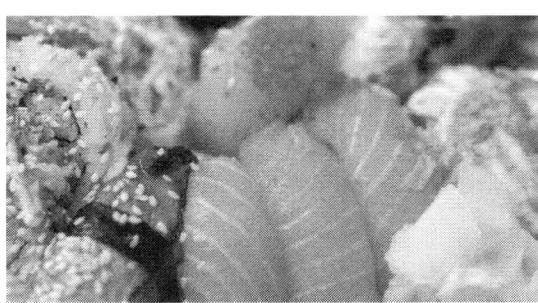

Intermittent Fasting is all about correcting the inherent problems in your body. The first thing it tries to improve is your insulin sensitivity. It is the single most important factor in weight loss and fat burning.

When your body is in a fasted state for longer than 10-12 hours the insulin level goes down. This is the perfect condition for burning fat.

You stop eating food for a certain period and create an energy shortage. It is not a slow supply of energy but a complete absence of it. In this case, the body comes in quick response.

Your body needs a regular supply of energy. The cells don't the individual capacity to store a lot of energy. However, they need a regular supply for running various functions. To provide energy in this case, the body starts using the energy reserves. The energy stored in the form of glycogen in muscles cannot be used by cells as this can only be used by the muscles where it is stored. But, the glycogen reserves in the liver can be used for providing energy to the body. In absence of regular energy supply, your liver breaks up the glycogen stores and starts providing energy to the cells. However, glycogen stores are not very high. If you follow a balanced lifestyle and keep practicing intermittent fasting the glycogen stores would be over very soon. This is the time your body would have no other option than to start burning the fat stores.

The absence of insulin in the blood during the fasting period signals the fat cells that the body is not in energy storage mode. Hence, using fat for energy becomes the only option. The major difference between the both is that dieting lowers the energy supply but the body still remains in the fat storage mode and insulin levels are usually high in the bloodstream due to frequent meals.

Intermittent fasting facilitates fat burning by reducing the insulin levels in the bloodstream. It paves the way for fat burning.

Without taking into consideration the role of insulin in the fat burning process, losing fat is very difficult. Once your body starts going through this feasting and fasting cycle it would start burning fat in routine. It is a reason people practicing intermittent fasting see a rapid decline in their waistline, thighs, and hips.

They not only lose their weight but also see a rapid decline in volume.

It is especially very helpful for women who have a strong desire to get in shape. Losing weight may be possible by several means but the fat bulges are the hardest to go.

Intermittent fasting is an easy and reliable way to get rid of these fat bulges.

The bulging fat in the body is only one part of the story and it may look bad but isn't that bad. The real problem is caused by the visceral fat in the body. It is the fat that starts to cover all your vital organs. It takes over your heart, liver, kidneys and affects their functioning. This fat is the hardest to burn. No kind of exercise or activity can melt away this fat. This nasty fat has the ability to impair the functioning of vital organs and may cause irreparable damage. Intermittent fasting is the only way to target this fat and get rid of it. If you want to remain healthy and fit burning this excess fat is the only option. The simple practice of Intermittent Fasting can help you in it.

Chapter 9:

Boost in Production of Fat Burning Hormones

Any help is a great help when it comes to fat burning. Losing weight is such an arduous task that people battling obesity would be ready to trade with anything. We may feel that whatever we may be doing only adds up to the weight but there are hormones that can help in shedding weight and fat really fast.

The Human Growth Hormone (HGH) is one such hormone that can help in cutting fat like magic. If you can unlock this hormone in your body, it will not only help you in losing fat accumulated at various places but will also make you look and feel younger and revitalized.

Little Bit About Human Growth Hormone (HGH)

HGH is a hormone that's linked to growth as the name suggests. Our body produces it in abundance when we are in our growth stage. This means the production of HGH is very high during childhood as the body formation and buildup is still going on. This hormone reaches the peak of its production during puberty. This is the reason kids grow really fast in their teens. Their body structure and appearance start to change dramatically. However, the production of HGH goes downhill one we cross teenage as most of the developing work is finished. Our body still produces this amazing hormone for usual wear and tear work.

Some interesting things to know about HGH production are:

- Our body produces HGH in sprouts. It means that there are periods in a day when the production of HGH can reach its peak.

- HGH production is high when you are in the sleeping state.

- HGH production becomes really high when you experience trauma or face accidents.

- For your body to produce HGH it must have high levels of Ghrelin the hunger hormone

- The levels of insulin should be the lowest in your body to facilitate the production of HGH as both have opposite jobs. HGH is a fat burning hormone and insulin is a fat storage hormone.

- HGH would accelerate the loss of fat and muscle building if you do exercise at the end of your fasting window. The presence of HGH in the body is very high.

- HGH is a very important hormone if you are trying to lose fat and build muscle mass. It prevents loss of muscle mass.

So, we understand that if our body starts producing HGH in ample quantity losing fat would become easier. The production of HGH gets lower as we age but it can be increased. We can reap all the benefits of HGH through intermittent fasting.

When we fast, our body fulfills all the conditions for the production of HGH. This will help in its production and if you add some exercise at the end of your fasting cycle, you can burn fat very fast.

The first condition of HGH production is that the insulin levels in your blood should be very low. After the last meal, it takes 10-12 hours for the insulin levels to go very low. This means that if you begin your fast around 6 in the evening, the levels of insulin would start getting low from 2. Your body will have ample amount of time to produce HGH as your first meal of the day would still be at least 6 hours away.

The second condition of HGH production is high Ghrelin level in the gut. It is a hunger hormone. Your gut keeps releasing this hormone after a few hours of your last meal. So, if you take your last meal around 6, your gut would start releasing the hunger hormone around 2.

The third condition states that the body should be in a completely rested state for high HGH production. In the wee hours of the morning, you would be in the rested state.

The fourth important condition is to exercise in the fasted state. It is important to note that you must exercise in a fasted state. If you consume anything with calories, the HGH levels in your body would go down. The exercise would still do its job but you will not get the added benefit of HGH.

This hormone works wonders in burning the fat deposits. If you want to burn fat then intermittent fasting and exercise can help you in unlocking HGH benefits.

Chapter 10:

Better Satiety

One resentment that many overweight people is that they are unable to control their desire to eat. They never feel full. They may like it or not but they can't stop eating. This adds to their weight and resentment too.

This may sound weird but this isn't appetite that leads to overeating but lack of satiety. It is a problem from which most obese people suffer and their obesity is the reason for this problem.

Our body has a perfect mechanism for everything. It signals various things through hormones that trigger the brain to do the things that it does. For inducing hunger and satiety also there are hormones. The hormone that induces the feeling of satiety or fullness after having a meal is called 'Leptin'. This is a very important hormone that signals your brain to stop eating.

Leptin is released by the fat cells to inform that the body's fat storage capacity is full and it needs to stop eating. The levels of leptin in your blood are the lowest when you are hungry and this level goes up as you eat. If you eat slow, you may start feeling full even after eating a small portion. This happens because your brain takes a while to recognize the leptin signal and trigger the feeling of satiety.

So, the leptin levels are the lowest when hungry and highest when full. The problem begins when there is inflammation in the fat cells. Excessive eating or continuous pressure to store fat can lead to this inflammation. However, the problem begins when there is an inflammation in the fat cells.

The inflammation causes the fat cells to keep releasing the leptin hormone at regular flow. It means that either you are hungry or full your fat cells would keep releasing leptin hormones at average flow. This constant bombarding of the leptin hormone makes the brain indifferent to the signal. There is no significant difference between the release of leptin in fasted or full state. Hence, the brain starts ignoring the leptin signals. It fails to signal you to stop eating as it keeps believing that you are still hungry.

This creates a serious problem of overeating. You not only add extra calories but also hammer your system with the same hormone.

More food means more energy storage and that would also mean more leptin release.

You can have excess food but there will be no satiety. You may feel full for a while but soon you would start feeling the need to eat again. This is not your hunger or the need to eat but simply a case of miscommunication of signals.

Intermittent Fasting can help you in a great way in this problem. The major cause of the problem is the constant release of leptin hormone. That gets accelerated by the fact that you keep taking meals at shorter intervals.

Intermittent fasting can ensure that your body has a longer period of fasting. During this period, there will be no intake of food. The inflammation of fat cells would still cause the release of leptin however the rate would be slow. As the pressure on the fat storage system eases with intermittent fasting the chronic inflammation would also go down. Your body would observe distinct periods when there is an absence of leptin and a high presence. This would again make the brain more sensitive to the signals.

So, intermittent fasting can help you in feeling fuller and satisfied. It would also help you in lowering your food intake by correcting the signals.

Intermittent fasting not only helps you in controlling your weight and cutting down of fat, but it also helps in improving all other important health biomarkers.
It can help you in controlling and reversing diabetes to a great extent. It can also lower chronic inflammation in your body that helps in curing many health problems. Intermittent fasting paves the way of autophagy. It is a process through which your body cleans itself of all the toxins and infections. It also helps in the regulation of various hormones.

The next few chapters will through some light on how intermittent fasting can help you in staying healthy and fit.

Chapter 11:

Help in Controlling Diabetes

Diabetes is one of the most common killers today. As per recent estimates, there are more than 110 million people suffering from diabetes and prediabetes in the US alone. This condition is spreading its wings all across the globe and even the countries with low-income levels are gaining on diabetes scale.

It is a debilitating condition where the patient becomes dependent on an outside supply of synthetic insulin. The doctors have been trying their best to control the menace but the best they have been able to do is find a way to manage the disease. There is no cure for this disease yet.

Intermittent fasting can help in this situation. There is a popular notion that synthetic insulin injections help in lowering high blood sugar levels. If we leave aside people suffering from Type I diabetes, most people do not have the problem of low insulin production. It means that the pancreas still produces the same insulin as it is required. It is the insulin resistance in the cells that leads to the problem. So, if a person can cater to the ssues causing insulin resistance, Type II diabetes can be reversed or at least easily controlled.

Intermittent Fasting Helps in Reducing Insulin Resistance
Insulin resistance is one of the biggest causes of the problem and we have discussed the ways in which intermittent fasting can help in reversing it. Intermittent fasting is the only way through which you can develop insulin sensitivity and beat diabetes or at least prediabetes.

Intermittent Fasting Helps the Pancreas by Giving them a Chance to Recover
Bad eating habits put a lot of pressure on the pancreas. The pancreas has to continuously pump insulin to lower the blood sugar levels. The pancreas produces various hormones like insulin and glucagon and also some enzymes. Putting the extra burden on the pancreas can lead to serious complications. If due attention is not paid on time it can create lead to the development of pancreatic insufficiencies. It can lower the ability of the pancreas to produce insulin and other hormones and enzymes.

Excessive fat and high cholesterol levels can also cause serious complications. If the triglyceride level in obese people remains consistently high as it usually is, it can even lead to pancreatitis.

Intermittent fasting can help you with both things. It lowers the load of continuously producing insulin hence your pancreas recovers from overload. Intermittent fasting is one of the best ways to switch to fat burning mode. In this, the body starts using triglycerides as the fuel to run various processes and hence excessive triglyceride levels also go down.

Helps in Reducing Weight

Excessive weight is always a problem with diabetes. The higher the weight the lower metabolic functions would be. Intermittent fasting helps you in fighting this weight issue and you are able to fight with the problem strongly.

Chapter 12:

Autophagy

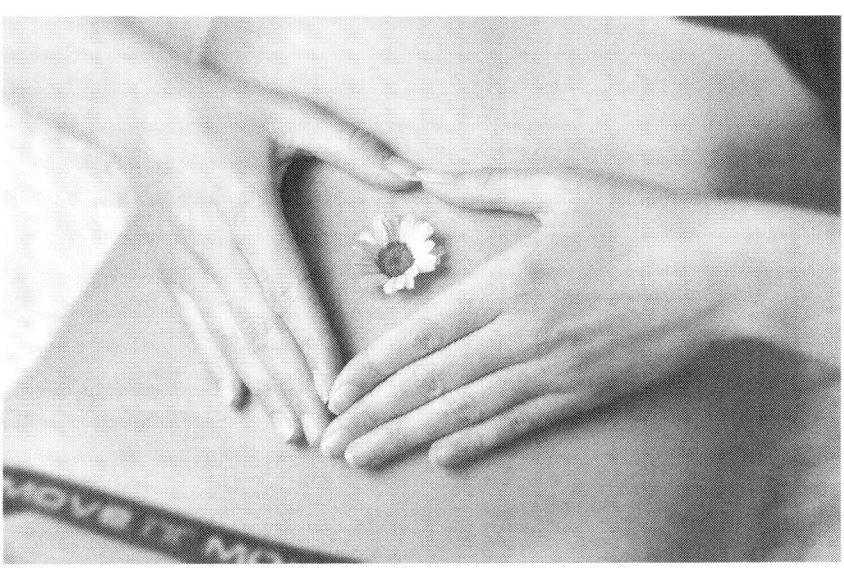

Autophagy is a relatively new concept the world is still trying to accept. However, our body has been using this phenomenon for millions of years. It is one of the most powerful ways to treat oneself that our body always knew. Autophagy is derived from

Greek which means 'self-devouring'. This is a sort of cleaning mechanism inside our body that can help in eliminating all kinds of toxins, germs, misfolded proteins, pathogens, bacteria. This process doesn't require any outside help and you can start feeling more energetic, relaxed, and relaxed once the process has taken place.

To begin with, A Japanese scientist by the name of Dr. Yoshinori Oshumi published his research on the topic in 2016 for which he was granted the Nobel Peace Prize. This research states that the body can purge all that clutter inside it once it feels that it needs to conserve the energy only for the most important purposes.

This means that if you fast long enough and in a proper way, your body can cure itself of most of the inflammations, infections, diseases, and disorders. When you starve yourself for long and the body starts to feel that it is not going to get energy supply any soon it can start the catabolic processes even at the macromolecular level.

This means that it will identify all the processes that are using misusing energy. For instance, the pathogens, parasites, fungi, mold, bacteria live inside us without giving back anything. When your body goes through autophagy it will identify all such life-forms and eliminate them.

In the same way, there are misfolded proteins, molecular waste inside our cells that keeps forming over time. When your body starts the purge it will identify all such misfolded proteins and recycle them to produce new cells and energy. This will not only clean your body but will also allow restrengthening.

Our body also identifies disorders, chronic inflammations, and diseases and starts eliminating them. All these problems not only make us ill but also use the energy of the body to make us ill.

When autophagy begins it starts eliminating all such processes. Chronic inflammations that have been troubling for years go away. It is one of the most powerful mechanisms for treating oneself. This process can stop the progression of many diseases that have been going on for years.

It has a very powerful anti-aging effect as it stops the processes that accelerate the signs of aging. Autophagy also has a very powerful impact on our cognitive function. It can stop the progression of neurodegenerative disorders and also reverse their effects. It implies that disorders like Alzheimer's and Parkinson's disease can be brought under control.

Autophagy also helps in promoting cardiovascular health, lowers hypertension, immunity problems, and chronic inflammation besides other issues.

This process can give you the boon of a rejuvenated life. You will have a new lease of life as your body gets the ability to heal itself. There is only one catch, autophagy can only begin in special circumstances. The first and foremost requirement for autophagy to begin is to experience acute energy shortage. This means that autophagy can only begin when your body stops getting any kind of energy supply and starts feeling that becoming efficient is the only way to survive.

Long fasting periods can induce autophagy. Once you remain in the fasted state for more than 36 hours, your body starts the purging process. However, this doesn't mean that you'll have to keep 36-hour fasts very often. Longer fasts are very effective in beginning the autophagy process, but intermittent fasting can also help you in getting its benefits.

There are two major benefits of autophagy:

It Cleans Your Body of Misfolded Proteins, Waste Cells, and Pathogens
Autophagy helps in cleaning your body of all the waste material that is not only making your body function inefficiently but also making you sick. The pathogens live inside your body and keep making you sick. They thrive on the energy of your body. Autophagy removes all these pathogens and paves the way to good health. The misfolded proteins and waste cells in your body keep your body cluttered. Autophagy not only cleans these misfolded proteins and waste cells but also recycles them. This gives your body new cells and also release a lot of energy that your body can utilize in the case of extreme energy shortage that it is going through.

Progression of Various Diseases can Slow Down
Autophagy is an amazing process that can slow down the progression of various diseases that can bring you down. Even ailments need the energy to spread in your body. For instance, cancer cells function like normal cells in the body. They thrive on the glucose energy supplied through food. If you undertake longer fasting and deprive your body of glucose energy, the progression of cancer can stop dramatically. Cancer cells can't spread on fat energy. So, if you start living on a fat diet and your body begins burning fat, the cancer cells can literally starve.

There are several chronic inflammations that thrive silently in your body because there is an abundant supply of energy. If you go on extended fasts, your body would start eliminating all these functions that are using up energy for inefficient purposes. Hence, chronic illnesses would cease to exist.

Studies have found that autophagy can also have a great impact on neurodegenerative diseases like Alzheimer's and Parkinson's Disease.
Several studies are currently going on to find innumerable health benefits of autophagy. This is a process that doesn't require anything extra to be done. You can simply induce autophagy by observing extended fasting in a correct and safe manner.
It is important that you understand that fasting for such long periods is not an easy task and it certainly needs a lot of practice and discipline.

Intermittent fasting can become your stepping stone for this process. Intermittent fasting in itself can give you the benefits of autophagy on a regular basis.
The next few chapters will explain the ways in which you can follow intermittent fasting and the correct way to do it for good health.

Chapter 13:

Intermittent Fasting - The Process

Intermittent fasting is a very simple concept. As the name suggests, it involves fasting for brief periods every day. We have already covered the health benefits it brings. This chapter will cover the things involved in the process.

The first and the foremost thing to understand is that 'Intermittent Fasting' is free and would cost you nothing at all.

So, even if you are concerned about the cost of losing weight this process is ideal for you. In fact, at the end of the day, it would help you in saving a bit of money. But, we'll get to that part later.

The second thing is, 'Intermittent Fasting' is easy. As the saying goes 'there is no free lunch in this world' intermittent fasting would also have its share of challenges.

However, as compared to other weight loss measures, following intermittent fasting is a cake walk. I consider dieting to be a much tougher thing to follow as it limits life to a great extent. Tough exercise routines are punishing and we have covered the stuff about pills and surgeries.

Looking at all other weight loss measures, intermittent fasting is the most charming kid on the block.

The third thing is, it has very limited chances of side effects and you will always have complete control of things. You can always change your intermittent fasting routine as per your convenience and still receive the benefits.

 It doesn't push you in a corner. It doesn't require intake of anything specific and hence the chances of side effects are very low. Of course, there are precautions to be taken. Like all procedures, not everyone can undertake intermittent fasting.
Women Who Need to Be Cautious are:

- It is not suitable for young kids or teenagers as they are in the growing stage and their energy requirements are high
- It is not suitable for women trying to conceive
- It is not suitable for lactating mothers
- Pregnant women shouldn't practice intermittent fasting
- The women with dietary issues or who are anorexic shouldn't practice intermittent fasting

- If you are under medication for some serious ailment like diabetes, hypertension, heart problems, you must consult your physician before starting intermittent fasting
- Women undergoing serious hormonal issues

These are all obvious reasons. Women undergoing pregnancy or nursing a child have the added responsibility of feeding another life. Their energy requirements are quite high. They shouldn't follow intermittent fasting.

One must always consult a physician before starting a new routine if he/she is under treatment for some serious illness.

Apart from the people falling under these categories, intermittent fasting is good for all.

What Would You Need to Do

Intermittent fasting doesn't change your life as you are living it. It simply asks you to make a few very simple and basic changes.

There are two main parts of intermittent fasting:

1. **The Fasting Window:** This is the time you will have to remain in the fasted state. It means that you can drink water and non- caloric beverages like unsweetened fresh lime, black coffee without sugar, unsweetened black tea, but can't have anything else in this window. Even the drinks advertised as zero calorie drinks are not allowed in this window. This window is usually longer as the main purpose of intermittent fasting is to give your system some rest and time to rejuvenate.

2. **The Eating Window:** This is the time when you can eat. Intermittent fasting doesn't put restrictions on the things you can eat. Therefore, you can eat pretty much anything in moderation. However, it is expected of a person trying to lose weight not to eat junk food or food items laced with a lot of sugar and carbs. The eating windows are comparatively smaller and hence too many meals may not be possible in this window. You will have to try to fit two to three meals in this window and eliminate snacks and frequent munching if you want to get the most out of your intermittent fasts.

You will need to follow the eating and fasting windows religiously. Some people have a habit of trying to have cheat days in everything. Once in a blue moon breaks are allowed even in intermittent fasting but that shouldn't be made a habit.

This is all you would need to do in basic when you practice intermittent fasting.

Intermittent fasting isn't some complex concept that needs to be taught. It is a life process we have been following naturally for hundreds of thousands of years. Wild animals still follow this practice. They eat once a day at the most and you very seldom find lions dying of heart attack or diabetes.

Intermittent fasting had been our way of life. It is a great way of life that can pave the way of health and wellness for you.

However, our ways have changed over the course of centuries. Therefore, again getting back to the roots can be difficult for many. We all fast for 6-8 hours at the least every day. Yet, extending that by another 4-6 hours can be a tough task for many. It would require preparation.

The next chapter would help you in preparing yourself for longer and somewhat tougher fasts and would show you the way ahead.

Chapter 14:

Preparation for Intermittent Fasting

Preparation is always very important when you start anything new. It keeps you in control and you don't feel lost and out of place. Although intermittent fasting is a simple and easy process yet food can be a big weakness for many.

Elimination of Snacks

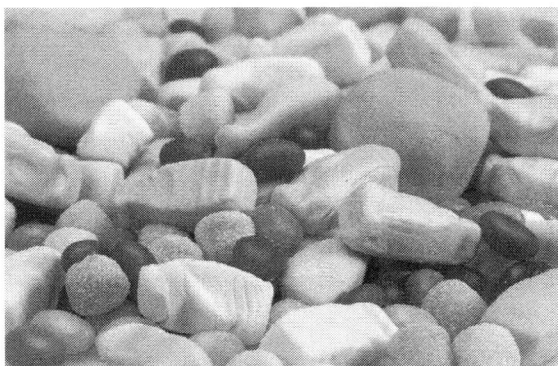

Before you begin intermittent fasting, it is important that you prepare your body for staying without food for extended periods. The first towards this is the elimination of snacks.

We may not realize it but snacks are our biggest enemies.

1.	They seldom contain anything nutritious

2.	They are full of sugar, salt, refined oil, and flours. All these things you will have to learn to avoid if you want to stay healthy and in shape

3.	They keep spiking your blood sugar levels frequently and load your system with empty calories

4.	They provide very little to your gut

On average, we snack for 3-5 times excluding the times when you are chewing gums, eating popcorns, drinking sodas and other such things although they also come in the category of snacks. The simple definition of snacking would be anything that adds calories to your system but gives very little to your gut. In fact, these snacks are more dangerous as they have a lot of sugar that not only launches too many empty calories into your system but it also leads to cravings. If you have a habit of eating sweet things in between your meals, you would find it really difficult to stay away from food. The sweets create a very strong food craving at short intervals.

Therefore, You will have to eliminate snacks from your daily routine. You can have your favorite tit-bits but that should only be along with your food.

It is important to understand that intermittent fasting doesn't restrict your calorie intake. You can consume calories within a reasonable limit. The calorie intake automatically goes down in intermittent fasting as your eating windows are short and hence this is not something on which you need to focus. Intermittent fasting is all about when to eat.

Start By 3 Meals a Day
You may be surprised that you may not be taking 3 meals a day even now. These are the times when we all are always running all the time. Most of us find it difficult to take out time to have 3 meals in a day.

Does that mean you are already practicing intermittent fasting?

The answer is negative. We may not have the time to take 3 proper meals but we take several improper meals within a day. Any kind of munching would be counted as a meal as far as intermittent fasting is concerned.

Therefore, you will have to start your day with a balanced but nutritious breakfast. Have a moderate lunch and finish off the day with light dinner.

The day you are able to sustain without any significant difficulty with these three meals, you will be ready for moving ahead with intermittent fasting.

Remember, intermittent fasting is no fad diet or trick that you can play on your body. It is a complete lifestyle change. Any serious lifestyle change would require your commitment. It isn't a trick that you have to pull off for a day. Therefore, you must only move ahead with the next step when you get really comfortable with your past routine.

Practice Any Routine for At least a Fortnight Before Moving to the Next
There would be times when you would feel that you are ready to move to the next step. There is always an excitement to see the change a more powerful process can bring. This excitement increases a lot more when you start getting results from the previous one. However, you must remember that intermittent fasting isn't a process that should be rushed.

Every intermittent fasting protocol has its own unique advantages. Even with 12-hour fasts, you would notice great changes in your life. But you must never rush the process. Always try to follow every protocol for at least a fortnight so that your body gets used to it. Once you get comfortable with that protocol then only you should consider trying the next one.

No Protocol is Superior
We all have mental preconditioning that the tougher the regimen would be the better the results. Although, this is correct to a great extent yet what we are looking here is individual capacity. Every individual has unique physical abilities. Trying to imitate someone else would be worthless. It is like expecting a fish to climb a tree. Some people will have excellent results by following a 12-hour protocol while others may get the same results by following a 24 hour fast. It all depends upon the individual. It is no competition and you must remember that the playing field is not even.

Therefore, your only consideration should be to find a routine that suits you the best. Don't go for the toughest, look for the routine that suits you the best.

Healthy Food Choices

Our food has a very important role to play in our lives. It has a direct impact on your health. Therefore, you must make healthy food choices.

Refined Sugar: Eating refined sugar can make your life difficult in fasts. It would create a lot of food cravings and you would always feel tempted to eat.

Refined Flours: Refined flours are bad for your gut and health. They are high on carbs and have very little fiber content. They will make you feel constipated and would make your life miserable. You should go for whole grains.

Refined Oils: Refined oils top the list of unhealthy food items. They are bad and full of unhealthy fat. You must always consume cold press oils like olive oil and coconut oil, peanut oil as they don't pass through any chemical process.

Deep Fried Food: Fried food contains a lot of refined oil as the restaurants will always keep their profit above your health. You must avoid deep fried things.

Avoid Carbonated Beverages: Carbonated beverages are bad for your health. They add a lot of empty calories to your system and confuse your gut. They are full of sugar and also cause cravings. You must avoid them.

Go for fresh food items. In place of fried food, choose baked or grilled food as it would be free of oil. Choose healthy fats and stay away from unhealthy fat and trans fat.

These are some simple tips that would help you in sailing through your intermittent fasting journey easily.

Chapter 15:

The 12:12 Fasting Protocol

This is the easiest fasting protocol and very simple in nature. If you are beginning intermittent fasting and have mastered the art of having only 3 meals a day then there is nothing difficult in store for you.

As the name suggests, this fasting protocol has a 12-hour fasting window and a 12-hour eating window. It is very easy to keep as most of the fasting window passes while you are sleeping. You would rarely feel the hunger pangs every.

However, being easy doesn't mean that this fasting protocol doesn't have health benefits. Fasting for 12 hours still gives your system great rest. The insulin resistance in the body would go down and you will also start losing weight.

The tough part in these fast is only to restrict yourself to 3 meals in a day.

The trick would be to have the three meals at equal intervals. This would help you in getting habitual of passing from one meal to another without having snacks.

There can be times when you feel a slight headache, uneasiness, or nausea in the beginning. However, there is nothing to worry as all these are primary symptoms of sugar withdrawal.

Our system has got habitual of frequent snacks and the glucose it gets from it. In the beginning, the body would try to adjust to the change. To ease the difficulty, you can always have water, unsweetened fresh lime or black tea or coffee. All these beverages don't add calories to your system and hence you can easily consume them. Try not to have too much caffeine as that can also make you feel uneasy.

You must follow this fasting protocol for at least a fortnight. You can also follow it for longer if you feel that your body needs a much longer time to adjust to the schedule.

Chapter 16:

The 16:8 Fasting Protocol

This is one of the most popular fasting protocols. It gives you great health benefits and it can easily become a part of your life. If you are looking for steady weight loss, fat burning and other health benefits with a moderate lifestyle then this is the intermittent fasting protocol for you.

It is the best routine for fast fat burning without facing the loss of muscle mass. This fasting routine accelerates your fat burning process while it causes the least amount of muscle loss.

In this fasting protocol, you will have to fast for 16 hours. The best time to begin fast is in the evening. However, if your work forces you to work late at night, you can also begin the fast before going to sleep.

For instance, if you go to bed early at night around 10, then you must have the last meal of the day before 7 pm. This will allow you at least 3 hours to digest your last meal.
 It would also mean that by the time you go to bed, you wouldn't be feeling hungry. Having the last meal of the day several hours before going to bed has several health advantages.

Your body gets proper time to digest the food. There is no extra pressure on your gut while you go to sleep and hence you will have a better sleep.

Around 2 am the insulin levels in your blood would be low and hence the production of HGH can also start. When you wake up around 6-7 your body would have ample storage of HGH. If you add even a little bit of exercise in the fasted state to your routine, you can have amazing weight loss benefits.

The ideal time to break the fast would be around 11 am. This is the time you will be having your first meal of the day before entering the most active part of the day. It is always best to have a healthy and balanced diet.

Your breakfast should have the right mix of fat, protein, and carbs along with the greens.

If you want to transition from one meal to another without feeling frequent hunger pangs, it is important that you keep the quantity of fat and protein high in your diet and carbs to the minimum.
The ideal ration of fat, protein, and carbs should be 70% fat, 20% protein, and 5% carbs in the form of whole grains and leafy greens.
Breakfast with this nutrient mix would keep you feeling fuller. Fat and protein don't make you feel hungry very fast.

Your goal should always remain to eliminate one meal from your day slowly and gradually. This means that you should always try to shift your one meal either it is your breakfast or lunch farther. This will ensure that you get two fulfilling meals and the time between your meals would also increase. This exercise is very important to ensure that your body experiences lest insulin spikes. It will work wonders in developing insulin sensitivity.

The lunch should be moderate. If it is too heavy you may not be able to have your dinner. The last meal of the day is important as after it you will be entering the fasting period. If you miss the dinner, it might get difficult to bear the hunger pangs.

Therefore, having a moderate lunch always helps the cause if you want to have it at all.

The dinner should be the healthiest meal of the day and it should be solely dedicated to your gut. It means you must consume the things that aid your digestion process.

You should try to have as much as leafy greens, fruits, and vegetables in dinner as possible. The best thing about leafy greens is that you don't need to worry about the quantity or ratio while having them. You can have leafy greens as much as you like.

The leafy greens provide essential vitamins, minerals, and nutrients. They also contain a lot of fiber that helps in keeping the digestive system healthy. They are good for your health and do not overload your system. The best thing about them is that they fill your stomach and ensure that you don't feel hungry for long. All these qualities make them an ideal thing to have at dinner.

This simple 16:8 intermittent fasting routine can ensure that you lose belly fat easily and also get healthy. Studies show that women can reduce 4-7% of their waistline by simply following this routine for 3-24 weeks. One very important thing to remember is that if you want to measure your progress, the ideal way would be to measure yourself with the tape. In this way, you will be able to measure the actual amount of fat you would have lost.

Weighing yourself on the scale may not be the right measure. This method helps in fat burning but it doesn't lead to loss of muscle mass in the process. On the contrary, you may even feel that you are getting some muscles. The fat is bulkier in volume but it weighs less whereas the muscles are compact but they weigh more. So, if you are losing the fat but gaining muscles, you may not lose any weight at all. However, you may be losing fat in good quantity and would be getting leaner.

Therefore, the right way to measure your progress would be through measuring tape.

This is an intermittent fasting protocol that can easily be made a part of life. The body easily gets used to this routine and you don't face any difficulty in following this routine in daily life.

So, if you want to burn fat and lead a healthy life, then you should follow this intermittent fasting protocol.

Chapter 17:

The 20:4 Fasting or One Meal a Day Fasting

As the name suggests, this fasting protocols are tough and involve longer fasting periods. Ideally, 20:4 fasting and One Meal a Day (OMAD) are similar in practice yet they have their own differences. OMAD routine involves eating the whole nutritional requirement in one meal. So technically, the fasting window can be as long as 23 hours.

The 20:4 fasting window also requires eating once a day but the eating window is bigger and you can stretch it for up to 4 hours. Effectively, you can also have two meals in this window with one small meal at the beginning and one large meal at the end of the eating window.

However, apart from this, both these routines are very similar in nature and the results they bring.

As you might already have guessed, these fasting routines are not for everyone. This routine is followed by people involved in competitive sports, bodybuilding, athletics, etc. These fasts increase the production of growth hormone a lot. Bulking muscles gets easier with these fasts.

However, these routines also require hard work. The fasts increase the production of HGH and other fat burning hormones. But, to build muscles, you will have to work very hard in the gym.

So, if you have an interest in such things and you are ready to work very hard, you can choose this intermittent fasting routine.
Here, it is also very important to note that keeping the 20:4 fasts is not very easy. Your body would never get habitual of this routine like the 14:10 routine which is very easy to make a part of a regular lifestyle.

In 14:10 intermittent fasting, the major fasting period passes away while you are still asleep. This ensures that you don't have to bear the hunger pangs for long.

This wouldn't happen in the 20:4 or OMAD. These fasting routines would be so long that you would be awake in the most difficult periods of the fast when the hunger pangs are the strongest.

Therefore, it is important that you choose these fasts keeping in mind your weight loss goals and sports aspirations. However, here it is important to state that these fasting routines have become a craze in the bodybuilding and sports community.

People are able to lose a lot of body fat through these fasts and gain muscles. These fasting routines have ensured that people get better results than most performance-enhancing drugs available in the market.

Chapter 18:

The 24 Hour Weekly Fasts

This version of fasting is tougher but followed infrequently. These are 24-hour fasts that you can keep once or twice a week on non- consecutive days. This intermittent fasting protocol requires you to remain in the fasted state for a complete 24 hours.

They are as difficult as they sound. Staying hungry for straight 24 hours is difficult. The thing that makes them even tougher is the fact that they are never a part of your routine. On any given day of the week, you begin your fast and then eat after 24 hours.

The most important part of this fasting protocol is getting off it. When your body has been in the fasting state for 24 hours, breaking the fast properly is crucial. It is important that one never breaks any long fast with a solid meal.

The longer food deprivation can cause problems in digesting solid food. One must break the fast with some warm liquid like soup.

It should be followed by some semi-solid food. This will not only nourish your system but also prepare your gut for the solid food. Once your system is properly nourished, you can eat solid food.

Another precaution to take on getting off a long fast is that one shouldn't overeat. The whole purpose of fasts is to reduce the load from your system. If you get involved in binge eating or impulsive eating after a fast, it would defeat the whole purpose of the fast.

These fasts are very helpful in detoxing your body and bringing healing effects. You can follow this routine once or twice a week.

Chapter 19:

Alternate Day Fasting or Eat-Stop-Eat

These fasts are also an extended version of the 24-hour fasting routine. The only difference between both the routines is that the 24-hour fasts are infrequent whereas these fasts can be kept as a routine.

The main principle is that one should keep 24 hours fasts on alternate days. It means you'll have one complete day of fasting and then another complete day of eating. Although these fasting routines are long, yet they have the potential to become a habit.

Alternate day fasts can be kept twice or thrice a week. They should only be kept on non-consecutive days of the week.

Although 24-hour fasts have a lot of benefits to offer, they can be really stressful, especially for women.

A woman's body is very sensitive to hunger signals. It has been designed in such a way that hunger is associated with insecurities. Long hunger bouts can throw the hormonal cycle of a woman for an erratic spic.

The reason behind this overreaction is the ability of a woman to give birth to a child. Only women have the ability to bear a child. Since the body hits puberty till it reaches menopause, a woman's body is always in the 'Ready Mode' to bear a child. Therefore, it always tries to keep itself aptly prepared.

It is very important for a woman to have adequate fat stores to bear a child. The body understands it and that's why it always clings to some extra fat. Food is also seen as a part of security. When women start fasting for very extended periods on a regular basis, there is always a risk of hormonal imbalance.

Therefore, it is always advisable to keep short fast if longer fasts are really not required for medical or health reasons. Longer fasts shouldn't be practiced simply for weight loss or fat burning.

Fat burning and weight loss impact can be achieved even by smaller fasts like 14:10 fasts or OMAD. The 24-hour fasting or alternate day fasting should only be practiced if detoxification or other health benefits like autophagy are sought.

Again, the important thing to remember about these routines is that entering feasting state properly is also as important as fasting. You will need to give your body the time to adjust to the change.

Another issue with longer fasting is that they are difficult. The best part about 14:10 fasts is that the most part of the fasting time is spent sleeping and hence women really don't have the hunger pangs. However, that isn't the case with longer fasts.

You may begin the longer fast at any time of the day or night, but you will have to spend most of the fasting time awake and experiencing the hunger pangs.

The best way to master this fasting type is to transition slowly. You must give yourself good exposure to smaller fasts before you move ahead with 24-hour fasts. Practicing shorter fasting routines first acclimatizes your body to these tough fasting routines and longer hunger pangs without disturbing the hormonal cycle much.

Women should also remember that they shouldn't practice fasts longer than 24 hours on a regular basis. Longer fasting schedules to induce autophagy should only be carried out only once in a few months. You should not undergo strenuous fasting without the consultation of your physician.

While fasting, women should also remember to drink a lot of water. It is important to keep yourself dehydrated to flush out the toxins. Water also keeps your hunger pangs low. Women can also rely on black tea and coffee to numb the hunger pangs during the fasting routine.

Chapter 20:

The 5:2 Fasting

This fasting routine has been included in the list despite the fact that in reality, it isn't fast. It is more of a calorie restrictive diet. However, studies have shown that this fasting schedule brings a lot of results for women and also doesn't affect their hormonal cycle at all.

Let us understand the 5:2 Fasting routine first.

The 5:2 mean that you will have to fast for 2 non-consecutive days of the week and you can eat normally for the other 5 days. Here, eating normally implies that you can have a healthy diet without consuming too many calories. This routine does require you to become calorie conscious.

On the fasting days, you must limit your calorie intake to 500 calories only or 25% of your usual calorie intake. This means that you will have to distribute 500 calories into the meals that you'll be taking throughout the whole day.

Women who have undertaken any form of dieting would sail through this fasting routine easily as it is very similar to dieting. However, the results are very different as the change in eating pattern forces the body to become more sensitive to insulin and leptin signals. Your insulin sensitivity would improve considerably and you would start losing weight from the very beginning.

It is a very relaxed type of calorie restrictive diet as you never feel very tempted to eat anything in particular because you always know that you can easily eat it the next day. This routine also helps you in staying away from the temptation of binge eating.

Chapter 21:

The Best Way to Incorporate Intermittent Fasting into Your Life

There are several things in this world that can be good for some, better for others, but worse for many. Practically, everyone has an individual good. There can be no generalization of the things that are good for everyone in most of the things. Weight loss programs aren't an exception in this.

The problem began when people started believing that what has worked for their neighbor or colleague would definitely work for them too. This doesn't happen in the practical world.

We all are individuals with unique body types and characteristics. Our bodies may react to the same stimuli in a different way. Some people may feel cold in a room while you may sweat. Their endurance levels may be the difference. While a person may start sweating like a pig after a short walk you may not even begin to perspire. All this happens because our bodies are different hence expecting the same results from a procedure would be amateurish.

In the same way, trying to imitate others is also an unwise approach. If someone you know feels comfortable with 24-hours fasts this doesn't put you in a compulsion to follow the same. You can get the same results by doing 14:10 fast and it would all depend on your body.

The real trick lies in understanding your own limits and respecting them. You have to remain confident in the results and keep working consistently towards it.
The beauty of intermittent fasting lies in the fact that it has the potential to become a lifestyle rather than a weight loss regimen.

The most important thing for the success of intermittent fasting routine in your life is to choose a protocol that suits your lifestyle the most and then to stick to it. Don't go for the best. Whatever protocol works for you will work the best in your life. It isn't the rigidity or toughness of the protocol that makes the difference. The discipline and dedication with which you follow it would matter the most in the end. Therefore, the most important thing is to stick to the basics and follow the routine. Choose a protocol that gels with your lifestyle. It may take you some time to find the best fit but there should be no rush. It is a lifestyle that you are going to choose for life. You can always devote some more time to finding it.
Pay attention to your food choices. Although intermittent fasting doesn't put a capping on the things you can eat, still it is always advisable to eat healthy things. Don't go for processed food. Try to stay away from refined sugar and things that have refined sugar. If you look closely, almost all the processed food items available in the market have refined sugar in varying proportions.

Food Choices

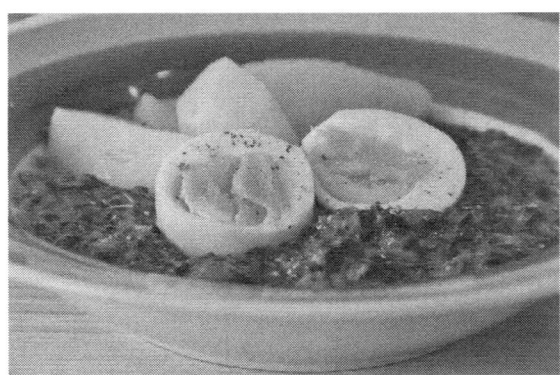

The best way to avoid refined sugar is to stay away from processed food or food items served by fast food chains. Even the salads served in most fast food chains are laced with so many dressings and syrups that they become unhealthy. The important trick is to return to the roots. Cook as often as possible. No one can cook better and healthier food than yourself. If you find cooking daily too much time consuming or you remain highly occupied for the whole week, you can prepare the food items once in a week, reseal and refrigerate them. This way you will be able to get healthy food in no time.

If you feel that you can't afford to take out the time for even this much cooking then think of the time it would consume when diseases bring you down. The pain, trauma, and setback it can have apart from financial and time-loss.

Sleep

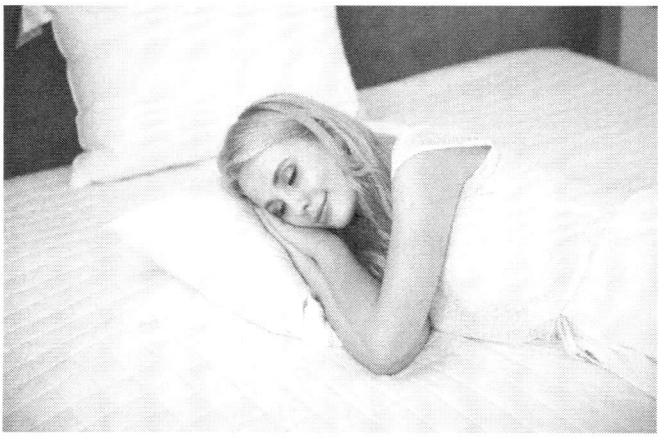

A healthy lifestyle would always be very important. We all have become so preoccupied with the race of life that we undermine the importance of simple needs in life. For instance, sleep is a very important requirement. Your body needs optimum sleep to carry out the most important functions. Yet, we all have started taking sleep for granted. We waste the nights in watching movies, drinking, parties, talking or working. If it isn't the utmost important, one shouldn't work at night. We aren't nocturnal creatures and we must act according to our circadian rhythm. If you are getting sound sleep at night, your body would be able to fight the weight better.

Your cholesterol and stress levels would also remain improved.

Intermittent fasting lays a lot of stress on giving the body the desired sleep. You must plan your day in a way that you can free up time for a good sleep. If you are observing longer fasts then you should specifically try to rest as much as possible. The body tries to recover in the fasting mode and hence putting a lot of pressure on it in such circumstances can be bad.

You must take proper rest and try to sleep early at night. Sleeping not only helps in passing the hardest part of fasting easily but it also allows the production of helpful hormones.

Exercise

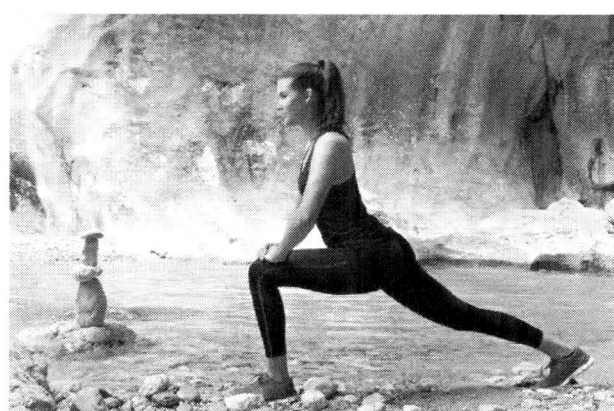

Exercise is very important for getting favorable results pretty fast. Intermittent fasting is a way to start burning fat naturally. Therefore, you will burn fat even if you keep leading a sedentary lifestyle. That's why this process is ideal even for the people suffering from morbid obesity and can't exercise. However, the results of intermittent fasting would get amplified if you indulge in High- Intensity-Interval-

Training (HIIT). HIIT ensures that you raise the energy requirement of specific muscles to a great degree in small sprouts. It doesn't put the muscles under chronic stress and also makes those muscles burn the energy stores. The HGH produced by the body during the fasting state also helps you in burning fat faster with the help of HIIT. This would make you look leaner and better while your fat burns.
A few important things to remember are:
You must not do HIIT daily. Do them on alternate days so that your body gets proper recovery time.

You should plan the HIIT on the days you are not in the fasting mode or immediately before you are going to break your fast. This is the time the HGH would be highest in your body.

Even if you are not able to do high-intensity exercise you should indulge in light exercises like walking, jogging, swimming, yoga, aerobics, etc.

All these activities also help in the metabolization of fat stores. The more active you remain in your daily life, the easier it would be to shed the extra pounds.

Light physical activities like walking can also help you in diverting your thoughts away from food. So, if you are feeling the hunger pangs and there are still some hours left of the fasting window, you should consider activities like walking that can divert from mind from food.

Routine

Intermittent fasting can only give you the best results when it is followed in routine. It means that you can't practice it once in a while and expect great results. In fact, if you try to do fasts in an irregular manner, you will face serious hunger pangs.

Our gut releases the hunger hormone called Ghrelin with great precision. It means that the gut can sense the usual time when you consume food and exactly around the same day you can feel the gurgling of the stomach. So, if you are keeping 14-hour fasts on a regular basis then after a few days you'll notice that you don't feel the hunger pangs before its time to break the fast. However, if you are not regular with the routine this wouldn't happen and you'd keep struggling with getting comfortable in a routine.

Making intermittent fasting a usual routine also helps in getting over the hassle of doing it consciously. After a bit of time, it would become a part of your life and wouldn't look unusual. This is the time when it would start showing the best results.

You would have a complete change in the way you lead your life and your overall health would start improving considerably.

Chapter 22:

The Ways to Deal with Problems and Side-effects

There are pros and cons of everything and intermittent fasting is no exception. It a complete lifestyle change and hence making the transition can be difficult for some people. This chapter would help in understanding the problems that you can face and how to deal with them.

While following intermittent fasting you can face mild symptoms like headache, cravings, hunger pangs, feeling of irritation, bloating, constipation, etc. if you are encountering such issues then there is no reason to worry as these aren't big or permanent problems. These issues occur because you are making a change in your lifestyle. There are remedies through which you can deal with these symptoms and soon they will subside.

Headache
It is the most common problem that people face. There is nothing to worry about the headaches as they occur when you are going through sugar withdrawal systems.

Our lifestyle has become such that our dependency on a carbohydrate-rich diet has increased a lot. We also keep consuming meals at frequent intervals and hence our body keeps getting glucose supply at short intervals. Our body loves glucose fuel as it is easy to burn and can be absorbed by the cells directly. However, being easy doesn't make it good. It leaves a lot of waste and residue in the body.

When you begin intermittent fasting, you block the regular supply of glucose fuel. Your body requires energy dump at short intervals. It can also derive energy from the fat stores but it is difficult to burn fuel and hence your brain starts giving you signals to eat frequently in the form of a headache. If you don't start eating frequently, your body would have no other option than to switch to fat fuel in the body. It is a clean fuel, leaves no toxic waste and residue. It would make you slimmer and also help in getting rid of diseases.

The easy way to counter the headaches is to have unsweetened black tea or coffee. These beverages help in dealing with the headache and also don't add any calorie to your system.

You can have them without breaking your fast.

Hunger Pangs

As we have already discussed in the book, the hunger pangs are a function of your biological clock. Even if you are feeling hungry it doesn't mean that you need to eat.

The feeling of hunger is created by the release of a hormone called Ghrelin. The gut releases this hormone at times when you have food in a normal routine. It means that if you are habitual of eating at 8 in the morning or you eat immediately after brushing, you would feel the urge to eat at these times. The ghrelin release is triggered by these signals. It wouldn't matter much that you had eaten a short while ago. The ghrelin release is also triggered by time and incidents and not just by hunger. Now, because the hunger pangs are more dependent on signals than actual hunger they can be shifted easily.

Another important thing about hunger pangs is that they are short. It means that if you are having hunger pangs, stomach cramps, and other such symptoms, you'll only need to hold on to it for a short while and they'll subside.

Diverting your attention toward other important things is also a good way to avoid hunger pangs.
Physical activities like walking, jogging, swimming, etc. can also help in subsiding hunger pangs.

If you must, you can also drink unsweetened fresh lime water, black tea or coffee without sugar or water to fill your stomach and it would also help in suppressing the hunger.

Very soon your gut would get used to the changed schedule and you would stop getting troubled by the hunger pangs.

Cravings

Cravings can mean a lot of different things for men but they have a completely unique meaning when it comes to women. Food cravings can arise in women due to emotional needs or psychological distress too. Women can find great solace in food, especially in sweets and desserts.

However, craving, in general, is bad and the biggest cause of food craving is the intake of sweets. Candies, chocolates, cookies, carbonated beverages and other such things that are high in sugar content can cause sugar cravings. One must always try to stay away from such things.

There are several reasons for that:
1.   These things add lots of calories to your system and it can be counterproductive when you are trying to lose weight
2.   Most sweets have very high sugar content and low fiber. Although these things would give a signal to your system that a lot of calories are coming, your gut would get nothing in reality. However, the release of digestive juices would be there. It would harm your system seriously.
3.   The more sweets you eat, the faster you'll feel the need to eat again. Refined sugar is more addictive than most addictive substances in this world.

4.   High sugar foods would make you feel fuller very fast but they would also make you feel empty stomach with the same speed. This is highly confusing for your gut and your blood sugar control system also remains engaged unnecessarily.

The best way to deal with this problem is to abstain from high sugar foods completely. If possible staying away from high carb food items is also highly advisable as they also have a lot of sugar. You must try to avoid processed food items as much as possible.

Eat food items that are high in healthy fats and proteins. The higher the fat and protein content in your food, the lower will be your food cravings and these nutrients take a lot of time to get processed in the gut. Your gut remains pleasantly engaged and is able to clean itself properly.

Frequent Trips to the Toilet

It is not very unusual for people to feel the frequent need to urinate when they begin their fasting routine. However, there is no need to worry as it is common for most weight loss programs. When you start any weight loss program and reduce your calorie intake, your body starts the protective mechanism.

It tries to lower energy needs. The water in your body apart from keeping you hydrated also helps in regulating the body temperature. However, as soon as you lower the calorie intake the body starts dumping the water to compensate for the energy deficit. But, there is nothing to worry as this is a temporary phenomenon and the water levels in your body would be back soon.

When you begin fasting your body also starts cleaning itself of the toxins and that also causes frequent urination. As long as you are not feeling any discomfort or the trips haven't increased a lot, it is not something that should worry you much.

You should keep drinking lots of water to compensate for the loss. If hypertension or other such medical issues are not there, you should even try having water with a pinch of sea salt. It helps in replenishing the loss of minerals that occurs due to excessive urination.

Felling of Irritation

One common issue that people can feel while beginning the fasting routine is a feeling of irritability. It isn't a permanent phenomenon and occurs only due to the fact that your blood sugar levels may fluctuate in the beginning. We have already discussed that your body may experience low blood sugar levels for extended periods and that is not a very bad thing if you are not suffering from some chronic problem like diabetes. However, low blood sugar can cause irritability as the body is frantically looking for energy.

This is the stage where even your body is learning through the transition phase. It is making the switch to the fat fuel when it doesn't want to. This is a temporary phenomenon that wouldn't last very long.

Heartburn, Bloating, and Constipation

Heartburn and bloating and common issues that you may face when you begin fasting. The reasons for bloating are simple, your gut keeps releasing the digestive juices at regular intervals but doesn't get anything to digest that causes the problem. However, this is a very temporary phenomenon as your gut would easily adjust to your new eating schedules and the problem would subside.

The heartburns are also part of the same process but they cause the most discomfort. The good thing is that they wouldn't last long. As soon as the release of digestive juices gets timed, bloating and heartburn would subside.

Constipation, on the other hand, can be a problem for many. The main reason for constipation isn't fasting but intake of improper food. It is a fact that your food intake may reduce when you begin

intermittent fasting as your number of meals go down. However, if you don't include high fiber food items in your meals, your gut wouldn't have much to process. This can cause constipation that may trouble you a lot.

The best way to avoid is to have fiber-rich food. Increase the salads and fiber-rich food in your meals and you would face no such issue. The important thing to remember is that you need to understand the problems you are facing and try to find the solution. Don't stick to a particular thing but try to find your best in the routine.

Intermittent fasting may become a big change in your life. You will have to make a few adjustments to welcome this change. It would be easy for you and even beneficial if you start making some adjustment to accommodate them. Don't be stubborn or a stickler for rules. Try to find your rhythm and flow with it.

Chapter 23:

Common Mistakes to Avoid

Intermittent Fasting is a great process that can bring exemplary health effects. However, any process can only work efficiently if its execution is right and silly mistakes are not done in the execution. This chapter will explain some of the common mistakes people make while following intermittent fasting. This chapter will focus on the basic mistakes that we make casually but which can harm our weight loss goals as well as health goals drastically.

Pay Attention to Macronutrients
This is one of the most important things to remember. The people who are suffering from obesity simply wants to get rid of this malice. They are ready to barter anything for it. They dream of a slender figure as the ultimate goal and this is where they become susceptible to make some of the most fatal mistakes.

Intermittent fasting or any form of dieting or calorie restrictive routine would put certain restrictions on you. Intermittent fasting doesn't put a cap on the amount of food you can eat or its type. However, that doesn't mean you can eat a lot. In most cases, you will have only 7-8 hours in reality to eat anything that you want. Although it may look a lot of time, you would find that the time for the final meal of the day approaches much before the previous meal has got digested. Missing that meal may mean that you'll have to go without food till the next meal. Therefore, the amount of food you can eat gets limited.

Other calorie restrictive routines put an explicit cap on the amount and type of food you can have. These things have a profound impact on your health. You may experience weight loss but that doesn't mean that you are getting healthy.
Your body can only get healthy when it is getting all the macro and micronutrients in the right quantity. It also needs vitamins and minerals. Getting all that while consuming limited calories can be difficult. If you don't pay proper attention here, you will end up with nutrient deficiencies.
You may get a slender frame but you will be battling with more problems than you started with.

The best way to counter this problem is to have a properly balanced diet. Intermittent fasting allows you a proper chance to do so as it doesn't put restrictions on quantity and types of food items you can have.The best way to pass this trick with qualifying marks is to have a very balanced meal. Your meals should be high in fat, moderate in protein and low in carbs.Before you begin to question the credibility of the suggestion, I would like to clarify some misconceptions:

Fat is not bad

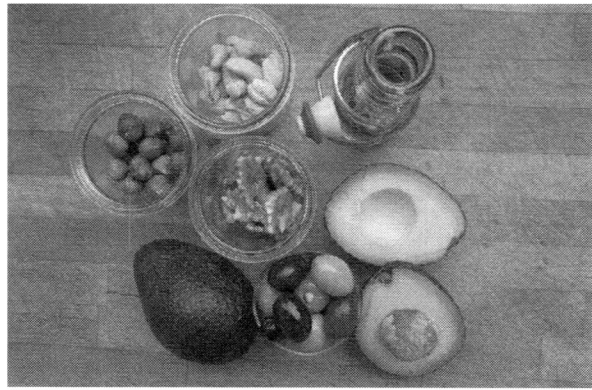

There is a popular misconception that eating fat is bad. Fat is the building block of life. It plays a number of important roles in our life. Our body can not function without fat. Fat, in general, is not bad. Trans fat or the poor quality fat that we get in processed food is bad. Fat in itself is a form of compact energy. Our body doesn't classify food as fat, protein, or cholesterol. Everything that you eat gets processed and is broken down as calories. This means that fat would also get converted to glucose, and so would happen with carbs. The benefit of eating fat is that you will be able to get more calories in a single meal in comparison to carbs.

Fat is very compact in nature and has almost double the number of calories per gram when compared to carbs. So if you get 8 calories per gram of carbs you'll get 16 from fat. Protein is also heavier and has more calories than carbs. This means that if you consume a high fat – low carb diet, you can get more calories. It also means that even if you have fewer meals in a day, you will not get energy deficient.

Fat should be consumed in greater quantities. You should select high-quality fat. The same goes for protein. You can get protein from animals and cereals and it would help you in muscle building and staying fit. The biggest advantage of having a high-fat, moderate protein, low carb diet is that it doesn't make you feel hungry very often. Fat and protein content in your meals would help you in transitioning from one meal to the other easily without facing the need to have snacks. Fat and protein-rich diets also contain a lot of minerals and vitamins. However, the highest part of minerals and vitamins and fiber should be obtained from carbs. You should consume a lot of leafy green vegetables, salads, whole grain foods. Leafy greens are bulky and but they do not weigh much. They don't add too many calories to your system but they provide most of the vitamins, minerals, phytonutrients, antioxidants and trace minerals required by your body. You can have leafy green vegetables as much as you want without worrying about calories. They are rich in fiber and hence keep your digestive system healthy and improve your immunity as well.

This is a part that you should never undermine in your pursuit to have a slender figure. If you ignore your health, the weight would come back faster than you can lose it. It will also have a very adverse impact on your health. You must always remember that you need to be healthy to fight weight and it isn't the other way around. The people who lose their weight drastically without a solid base are called sick and not healthy.

You must never forget the macronutrients in your meal as they would become the pillars of your health.

Don't Get Greedy in the Feasting Windows

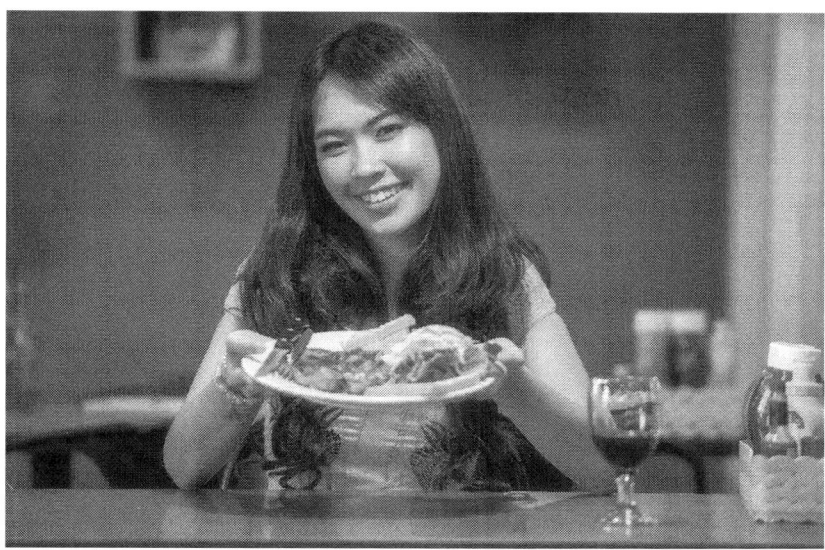

Food has its own temptation. It looks like the most alluring thing in the world when you have been deprived of it for a long time. This would happen with you too. But, it is important that you don't get greedy at such times and lose control. It is very important that you get off your fasting windows in a proper manner.

The biggest mistake people make is they eat a lot after breaking their fast. This can cause several problems and poor digestion is one among them. In the fasting state, the gut gets to stay away from food for extended periods and hence it can get a bit dry. Stuffing it with heavy food can cause problems. The best way to begin the day is to start with liquid food and then transition to semi-solid and solids.

You should also mind the quantity of food that you eat. Our brain takes much longer to understand the leptin signals that you are full. By the time your brain tells you that you are full, you would have already overeaten. The best way out is to either eat slowly as this would give your brain the time to assess your satiety levels. You can also stop eating when you feel that you are 80% full. Generally, by this time you would have eaten your fill. If you want to test this, you can wait for sometime after feeling 80% full and you'd find that you are no longer feeling hungry. It happens as the fat cells are able to properly communicate to the brain that it doesn't need to eat anymore.

Don't Try to Rush the Process

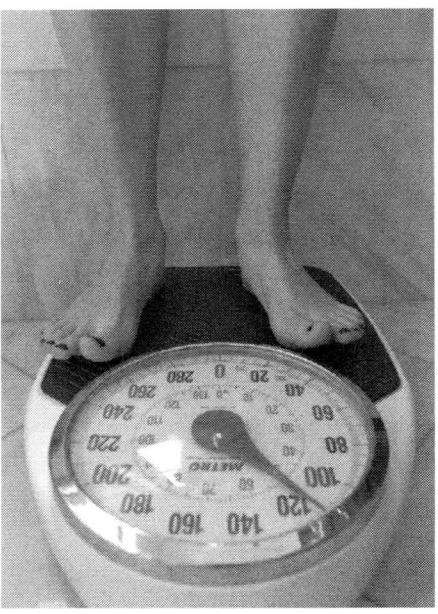

Slow and steady wins the race. This is an adage we all have heard but most of us fail to believe. We want quick results and for that, we are ready to make the jumps. However, this is not how the body works. Your body makes the transition very slowly. It needs the time to adjust to any kind of change positive or negative and the same would happen even in case of intermittent fasting.

If you want to succeed with the process you must ensure that you stick to every stage for some time. You must give your body the required time to adjust. There would be decades old habits that would need to change and it can be difficult for your body at times. If you want your body to react favorably to the change, you must not rush the process.

Fasting in men and women is completely different. Men have a very rugged system and it doesn't get affected by a bit extended fasting schedule. However, it isn't the case with women. If you try to jerk your system a bit harder, it can affect your health adversely. Your hormonal system may go for a spin and it may take very long for it to normalize. A woman's body reacts very differently to stress signals and hence caution and patience are essential.

Start with the easiest process and give your body the time to adjust to the small breaks. Once it gets used to a certain amount of brake, try to extend it a bit slowly. Don't do anything very fast. Always go step by step and you will get your goal easily and without unnecessary difficulties.

Perseverance is the Key

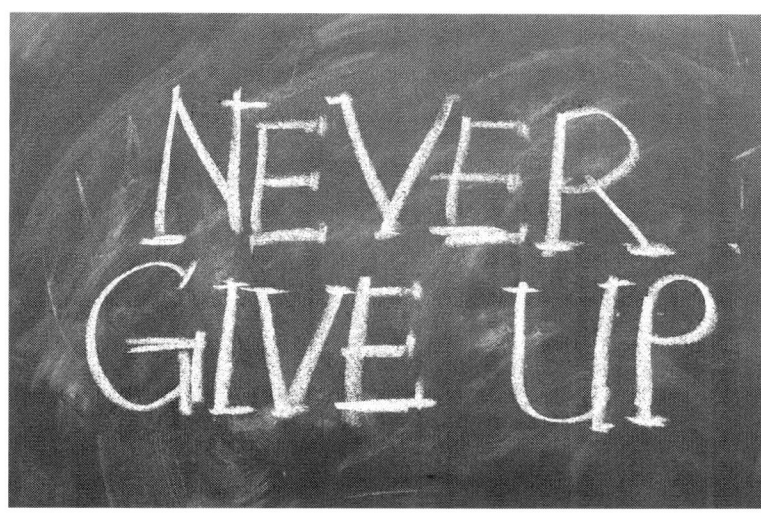

Impatience is a big problem in people battling with weight. There is no fault of theirs as they are already under great pressure. Most people trying to lose weight have already faced disappointment with other weight loss measures and hence they want to see the results fast to believe them. They are not ready to wait very long to get the results.

This is a point where problems can occur. Intermittent fasting is not any wonder- process. It is a wonderful process but it doesn't work by magic. It tries to correct the problems that may have reached their current state of development in decades at least.

It would take some time for the results to come. You will have to work patiently and not lose hope while the results come. If you quit in between, you wouldn't be able to know if you were making any progress or not. It isn't a process that works overnight. It would require you to take the leap of faith and invest your time and energy into it.

Don't Frame Unrealistic Expectations

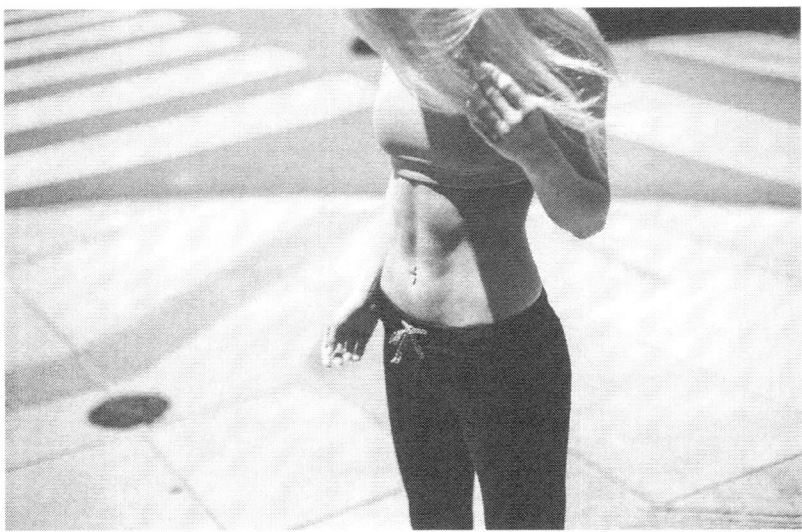

We all like to dream big and that is a good thing. However, we must also remain grounded in reality. This will help in accepting the facts and save a lot of disappointments. Many times we are so engrossed with the imaginary expectations that we fail to recognize the gifts we get. If weight loss is your goal then think of the amount of time you are ready to devote, the lengths to which you can go for it and the medical conditions you are facing. Without considering all these facts, expecting a complete makeover would be absurd. If you have made such expectations then you will not even be able to enjoy the weight loss you are observing. Your expectations would overshadow the results. It is important that you remain realistic.

Properly Manage Your Fasting Time

It isn't unusual for some people to mismanage their time. Most of us do it in our daily lives. However, poor management of the fasting time can be a cause of great distress for you. It can make your weight loss journey difficult and painful. You cannot remain thinking about food all the while you are in the fasted state. This would create problems for you and your gut would also remain confused. The best way to manage the fasting time is to keep yourself busy. The last leg of your fasting window should always be planned in such a way that you remain aptly engaged. The idler you are the higher are the chances that you'll only think about food.

Engaging in heavy physical activity is one of the best ways to put off hunger. The hunger in today's age is a highly psychological phenomenon. Our bodies have ample energy stores to run without food for months. It is our mind that is always drawing us towards food. You only need to stall it for a few hours. Walking, running, laughing, talking to friends, engaging in serious discussions are some of the ways through which we can stall hunger and remain unaffected.

These are some of the common mistakes that we make and which can mar the results we get. Intermittent fasting is a very simple and easy way to lose weight. It doesn't require much of your time and effort. You only need to make up your mind once and bring it into your life. Even if you are following any other weight loss measure, intermittent fasting can still fit into your lifestyle.

Chapter 24:

Tips to Stay Motivated

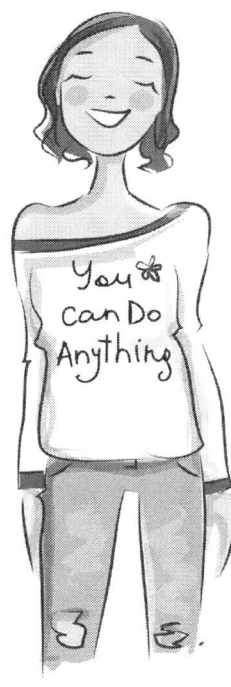

Losing weight isn't an easy task especially for women. It also becomes a lot difficult as there are stigmas attached to the weight. Most obese or overweight people also find that their own body doesn't support them in weight loss efforts. There are medical conditions attached that make losing weight even more difficult.

However, the efforts must continue as excess weight is simply not a cosmetic problem. It is also bringing you down firmly. Obesity comes as a complete package of diseases. It slows down your defense mechanism. You start feeling that nothing is going in your favor.

The things start turning ugly when some of your weight loss attempts fail. There is an internal sense of failure and in some cases, there is outside ridicule too. People stop trying in fear of failing. They start considering poor health a better option than failure.

If someone is in such a mental or emotional state, no weight loss measure can help. Losing weight is simply not a physiological effort but a mental one too. It is important that you stay motivated throughout your weight loss journey. You must find your pillars of strength the people towards whom you can look up to in times of distress. There will be times when you will feel low, broken, failing or distraught, there should be someone to whom you can confide and share your feelings. But, apart from everyone else, it is important that you remain firm on your ground. It is important for you to remain positive. There are some ways through which you can remain positive throughout the journey.

The biggest push is only needed in the beginning before you have achieved any result. Once you start getting results and clear the milestones, your success would be your motivation.

To remain motivated in the early stage you can seek the following ways.

Take Help of Positive Affirmations

Positive affirmations are very inspiring. They fill us with positive energy and help in clearing away negative thoughts. You can read positive affirmations, listen to them on the internet or recite them loudly. They help in every way. Positive affirmations keep your mind clear and give you the energy to sail through the bad times. They don't take much of your time and you also don't have to remain dependent on others.

Taking help of positive affirmations is a great way to remain motivated.

Share Your Goals with Your Family and Friends

Sharing such things with others is always difficult. There is always the fear of being judged on the results. However, there are always some people in everyone's life who don't judge. It can be your parents, partner, siblings, or close friends. Share your goals with them and the problems you are facing in the way. Discuss with them the ways to get out of the problems. They can give you suggestions or at least lend their ears. Even letting it off your chest is also a great relief most of the times.

You will always have an assurance that there are people who really understand your efforts and are supporting you in them. It is not necessary that you disclose your goals to everyone but sharing it with some of your very close people is always a good idea.

Professional Help

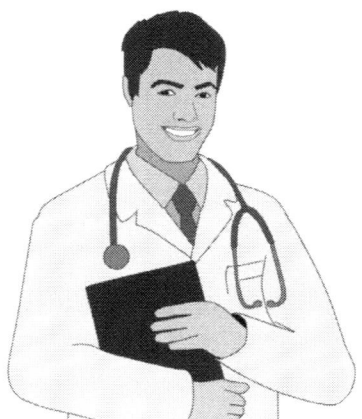

Obesity is not a rare problem these days. In fact, it is one of the most common ailments faced by people. Therefore, you can also get several professionals with whom you can discuss your problems and progress. You can consult your doctor and periodically discuss your progress. This serves two purposes. First, there will be a professional to guide you about the progress. You will get professional opinions on time about the problems you face on your way. You can get tips on nutrition and also advice about the ways to improve the progress.

Support Groups

It is a cost-effective way to get help. Support groups can emerge as pillars of strength. There are many people suffering from the same problems. They are also going through the same trials and tribulations. They can prove to be a great help in case you need moral or mental support. Most of the people in support groups are facing similar problems and hence your problems can be common. You can get the tips that worked for them. Such support groups can be of great help.

Keep the Atmosphere at Your Home Conducive

Most of the times our surrounding atmosphere also makes our efforts difficult. For instance, if your fridge is full of carbonated beverages, fast food snacks and munchies, it would be difficult to control the urge to eat. If people in your home are casually eating things all the time, you would start feeling punished and left out. It is important that you explain your goals and make arrangements so that the process gets simpler and not difficult.

It is important that you clear your fridge. If it is shared by others then you should limit your access to the fridge.

Your kitchen should be stacked with healthy things and junk food should be removed so that you don't get tempted or excuse to eat them.

Remove all kinds of sweets and chocolates from your home. They are irresistible and can break your will in your weak moments.

By thinking of losing weight you have already cleared the first hurdle. You only need to become more conscious of your choices to succeed in your efforts.

Chapter 25:

The Keto Diet Plan for Intermittent Fasting – How to accelerate your weight loss

The keto diet will set up your body to deplete the stored glucose. Once that is accomplished, your body will focus on diminishing the stored fat we have saved as fuel. The new technique will begin with 5% for carbs, 75% fats, and 20% for protein daily. Many people don't understand that counting calories don't matter at this point since it is just used as a baseline. Your body doesn't need glucose, which causes these 2 stages:

- *The Stage of Glycogenesis:* The excess of glucose converts itself into glycogen, which is stored in the muscles and liver. Research indicates that only about half of your energy used daily can be saved as glycogen.

- *The Stage of Lipogenesis:* If there is an adequate supply of glycogen in your liver and muscles, any excess is converted to fat and stored.

Your body will have no more food (much like when you are sleeping), making your body burn the fat to create ketones. Once the ketones break down the fats, which generate fatty acids, they will burn-off in the liver through beta-oxidation. Thus, when you no longer have a supply of glycogen or glucose, ketosis begins, and the consumed/stored fat will be used as energy. The Internet provides you with a keto calculator at "keto-calculator.ankerl.com." Begin your process by making a habit of checking your levels when you want to know what essentials your body needs during the course of your dieting plan. You will document your personal information, such as height and weight. The Internet calculator will provide you with essential math.

When the glycerol and fatty acid molecules are released, the ketogenesis process begins, and acetoacetate is produced. The Acetoacetate is converted to two types of ketone units:

- *Acetone:* This is mostly excreted as waste but can also be metabolized into glucose. This is the reason individuals on a ketogenic diet will experience a distinctive smelly breath.
- *Beta-hydroxybutyrate or BHB:* Your muscles will convert the acetoacetate into BHB, which will fuel your brain after you have been on the keto diet for a short time.

You will discover how flexible the ketogenic methods are when coupled with the intermittent fasting techniques. You will lose weight differently with each method, and other people may not have the same goals as you.

For now, as a beginner, you will begin by using the first method, as shown below. This is an important step; you must decide how you want to proceed with your diet plan. It is always best to discuss this essential step with your physician.

These are the four methods, for you to understand the different levels of the keto diet plan better:

Keto Method # 1: The standard ketogenic diet (SKD) consists of high-fat, moderate protein, and is low in carbs.

Keto Method # 2: Workout times will call for the targeted keto diet, which is also called TKD. The process consists of adding additional carbohydrates to the diet plan during the times when you are more active.

Keto Method # 3: The cyclical ketogenic diet (CKD) entails a restricted five-day keto diet plan, followed by two high-carbohydrate days.

Keto Method 4: The high-protein keto diet is comparable to the standard keto plan (SKD) in all aspects. You will consume more protein.

Macro Guidelines

Ketogenic 0-20 Carbs Daily: Generally, this low level of carbs is related to a restrictive medical diet, where the patient is restricted to 10 to 15 grams each day to ensure the proper levels of ketosis remains. The Charlie Foundation is one of the plans used to promote the treatment of epilepsy.

Moderate 20-50 Daily Carbs Allowed: If you have diabetes, are obese, or metabolically deranged, this is the plan for you. If you are consuming less than 50 grams daily, your body will achieve a ketosis state, which supplies the ketone bodies.

Liberal 50-100 Daily Carbs Allowed: This option is best if you're active and lean and are attempting to maintain your weight.

Calorie Counting Versus Micros

The short of counting calories is that they don't tell the whole story. You can fill up on the "right" calories, and you may also lose muscle mass. For example, you count one hundred calories of avocado (a fat), which is better than one hundred calories from a cookie (carbs). That is why keto counts the macros (fat, protein, and carbs), not the calories.

Remember This Formula: You will need to calculate your net carbs on some of the recipes you discover on the Internet; some list only the total carbs. If that happens, just take the total carbs listed (-) fiber (=) the total net carb, which is what you need to track an accurate count, so you can remain in ketosis.

Foods Included in the Intermittent Fasting Plan

Fresh Vegetables

You need to add plenty of veggies to your lunch or dinner menu plans. Each of these has the Net Carbs listed per 100 grams or 1/2 cup serving:

- Alfalfa Seeds – Sprouted – 0.2
- Arugula – 2.05
- Asparagus - 6 spears – 2.4
- Hass Avocado – ½ of 1 – 1.8
- Bamboo shoots – 3
- Beans – Green snap – 3.6
- Beet greens – 0.63
- Bell pepper – 2.1
- Broccoli – 4.04
- Cabbage – Savoy – 3
- Carrots – 6.78
- Carrots – baby – 5.34
- Cauliflower – 2.97
- Celery – 1.37
- Chard – 2.14
- Chicory greens – 0.7
- Chives – 1.85
- Coriander – Cilantro leaves – 0.87
- Cucumber with peel – 3.13
- Eggplant – 2.88
- Garlic – 30.96
- Ginger root – 15.77
- Kale – 5.15
- Leeks – bulb (+) lower leaf – 12.35
- Lemongrass – citronella – 25.3
- Lettuce – red leaf – 1.36
- Lettuce – e.g., iceberg – 1.77
- Mushrooms brown – 3.7
- Mustard greens – 1.47
- Onions – yellow – 7.64
- Onions – scallions or spring – 4.74
- Onions – sweet – 6.65
- Peppers – banana – 1.95
- Peppers – red hot chili – 7.31
- Peppers – jalapeno – 3.7
- Peppers – sweet – green – 2.94
- Peppers – sweet – red – 3.93
- Peppers – sweet – yellow – 5.42
- Portabella mushrooms – 2.57
- Pumpkin – 6

- Radishes – 1.8
- Seaweed – kelp – 8.27
- Seaweed – spirulina - 2.02
- Shiitake mushrooms – 4.29
- Spinach – 1.43
- Squash – crookneck – summer – 2.64
- Squash – winter – acorn – 8.92
- Tomatoes – 2.69
- Turnips – 4.63
- Turnip greens – 3.93
- Summer squash - 2.6
- Raw watercress - 3.57
- White mushrooms – 2.26
- Zucchini – 1.5

Chili Peppers: The chemical found in chili peppers is called capsaicin, which will boost your metabolism. The capsaicin will increase the fat and calories you burn during your intermittent fasting plan. Twenty research studies indicated that you would lose/burn approximately fifty extra calories daily. However, all researchers now agree with the theory. At any rate, enjoy the chili peppers.

Fresh Fruits

It is essential to eat plenty of fruits while on the ketogenic diet plan. Enjoy these according to your daily limits of carbohydrates. This collection of keto fruits are 100 grams each for each 1/2 cup serving:

- Apples – no skin, boiled – 13.6 total carbs
- Apricots – 7.5 total carbs
- Bananas – 23.4 total carbs
- Fresh Blackberries – 5.4 net carbs
- Fresh Blueberries – 8.2 net carbs
- Fresh Strawberries – 3 net carbs
- Cantaloupe – 6 total carbs
- Raw Cranberries – 4 net carbs
- Gooseberries – 8.8 net carbs
- Kiwi – 14.2 total carbs
- Fresh Boysenberries – 8.8 net carbs
- Oranges – 11.7 total carbs
- Peaches – 11.6 total carbs
- Pears – 19.2 total carbs
- Pineapple – 11 total carbs
- Plums – 16.3 total carbs
- Watermelon – 7.1 total carbs

Excellent Spices

Black Pepper: Pepper promotes nutrient absorption in the tissues all over your body, speeds up your metabolism, and improves digestion. The main ingredient of pepper is <u>alkaloid piperine,</u> which gives it the pungent taste. It can boost fat metabolism by as much as 8% for up to several hours after it has been ingested.

Basil: (1 whole leaf, 0.5 gram is <u>0 net carbs)</u> You can use fresh or dried basil to maximize its benefits. Its dark green color is an indication that it also maintains an outstanding source of magnesium, calcium, and vitamin K, which are excellent for your bones. It also helps with allergies, arthritis, or inflammatory bowel conditions.

Cinnamon: (1 tsp. is <u>0.6 grams net carbs</u>) Use cinnamon as part of your daily plan to improve your insulin receptor activity. Just put one-half of a teaspoon of cinnamon into a smoothie, shake, or any other dessert.

Raw Ginger Root is <u>*0.9 net carbs*</u> *for 1 tbsp and involves* over 25 antioxidants. It maintains hefty anti-inflammatory elements to help reduce muscle aches and the pain and swelling of arthritis. Ginger is best known for its ability to reduce nausea and vomiting and its soothing remedy for sore throats from outbreaks of flu and colds. Have a tea made with hot water simmered with a small amount of lemon and honey and a few slices of ginger as a soothing tonic when you're sick.

Cumin Powder: (1 tbsp. is <u>2 grams net carbs</u>) Cumin maintains abundant antioxidants which are excellent for your <u>digestion</u> and so much more. It also stimulates the pancreas and gallbladder to secrete bile and enzymes which work to break down the food into usable nutrients your body needs to function healthily. Cumin also helps detoxify the body and is beneficial for several respiratory disorders, including bronchitis and asthma. Cumin is also an excellent source of vitamin A & C, as well as iron, which are all excellent for your immune system.

Cloves: Cloves possess a spicy and sweet flavor, but they also contain powerful natural medicine, including strong antiseptic and germicidal components that can help ward off arthritis pain, gum and tooth pain, and infections. They also relieve digestive problems.

Acceptable Sweeteners

Swerve Granular Sweetener is an excellent choice as a blend. It's made from non-digestible carbs sourced from starchy root veggies and select fruits. Start with 3/4 of a teaspoon for every one teaspoon of sugar. Increase the portion to your taste.

Stevia Drops offer delicious flavors, including hazelnut, vanilla, English toffee, and chocolate. Some individuals think the drops are too bitter, so use only three drops at first to equal one teaspoon of sugar.

Xylitol is at the top of the sugar alternatives, which is an excellent choice to sweeten your teriyaki and barbecue sauce. Its naturally occurring sugar alcohol has a glycemic index (GI) standing of 13.

Beverage Options

Coffee: Your caffeine levels can help increase the metabolic rate by approximately 11%. Studies have shown consumption of a minimum of 270 mg of caffeine—about three cups of coffee—will burn away an additional 100 calories daily. The rates can surely boost your intermittent fasting, as long as you leave it sugar-free.

Tea: Tea is offered as a good source of beverage because of the catechins in the tea conglomerate with the caffeine to help speed up your metabolism. The catechins are an antioxidant and a type of natural phenol which is from the chemical family of flavonoids.

An additional 100 calories can be burned daily to increase your metabolism by four to ten percent with the use of green and oolong tea. The effects may be different with each fasting participant.

Include Healthy Fats & Oils

Extra-Virgin Olive Oil (EVOO): Olive oil dates back to centuries, back when oil was used for anointing kings and priests.

High-quality oil with its low acidity makes the oil have a smoke point as high as 410° Fahrenheit. That's higher than most cooking applications call for, making olive oil more heat-stable than many other cooking fats. It contains (2 tsp.) -0- carbs.

Monounsaturated fats, such as the ones in olive oil, are also linked with better blood sugar regulation, including lower fasting glucose, as well as reducing inflammation throughout the body.

 Olive oil also helps prevent cardiovascular disease by protecting the integrity of your vascular system and lowering LDL, which is also called the "bad" cholesterol.

Coconut Oil: You vamp up the fat intake with this high flash-point oil. Enjoy a coconut oil smoothie before your workouts.

Use it with your meats, chicken, fish, or on top of veggies. It will quickly transfer from solid form to oil according to its temperature.

Other Monounsaturated & Saturated Fats

Include <u>these</u> items (listed in grams):

- Avocado, Sesame, Olive, & Flaxseed Oil – 1 tbsp. – 0– net carbs
- Olives – 3 jumbo – 5 large or 10 small – 1 net carb
- Chicken fat, Beef tallow & Duck fat – 1 tbsp. – 0 net carbs
- Unsweetened flaked coconut – 3 tbsp. – 2 net carbs
- Ghee & Unsalted Butter – 1 tbsp. – 0 net carbs
- Egg yolks – 1 large – 0.6 net carbs
- Organic Red Palm oil – e.g., Nutiva - 1 tbsp. – 0 – net carbs
- Various Dressings
- Keto-Friendly Mayonnaise

Other Choices for the Ketogenic Plan

- *Grass-Fed Butter:* You can promote fat loss with butter that is almost carb-free. The butter is a naturally occurring fatty acid which is rich in conjugated linoleic acid (CLA). It is suitable for maintaining weight loss and retaining lean muscle mass.
- *Ghee* is also a great staple for your keto stock, which is also called clarified butter.
- *Yogurt:* Coconut milk is easily digested and contains fats, including lauric acid. Yogurt provides transient bacteria since it feeds existing healthy gut bacteria as they pass through your intestinal tract.

Include These Cold Items

- Full-fat sour cream
- Goat cheese
- Full-fat cream cheese
- Parmesan cheese
- Hard & soft cheeses, e.g., mozzarella or sharp cheddar

Chapter 26:

How to Get Started on the 16/8 Plan

You will still be able to enjoy your regular meals, except you are eating in the eight-hour window.

How to Begin

Step 1: Choose a non-stressful week to begin the ketogenic diet plan.

Step 2: Purge the pantry and fridge.

Step 3: Restock the fridge and pantry with ketogenic food items.

Step 4: Consider skipping one meal each day. Maybe sleep a little longer and have brunch.

Step 5: Initially, don't exceed your net carbs and don't limit the fat and protein you consume.

Step 6: Make a routine. Drink a large glass of water and have a supplement of a ½ teaspoon of MCT oil or 2 teaspoons of coconut oil.

Step 7: Keep track of your ketone levels.

Once you have set your goals and calculated how many carbs you are allowed in one day, it is time to explore the Lean-Gains Method fully.

The 16/8 Method is also called the Lean-Gains Method. The plan is used as a routine targeted explicitly for the removal of body fat and to improve lean muscle mass. One of the most noteworthy benefits of this type of fasting is that it's incredibly flexible so that it will work well if you have a varied schedule. This safe program provides a fasting window of 16 hours, with hours of eating at 8 hours. The easiest way to attempt this schedule is to stop eating after dinner in the evening and wait 14 hours, which means skipping breakfast and picking things up in the early afternoon. For women, you'll fast for 14 hours compared to 16 hours for men before allowing a reasonable quantity of calories for the remaining 8 to 10 hours. Most people find it helpful to either eat two large meals during the 8 or 10-hour feeding period or split that time into three smaller meals since that is the way most people are already programmed.

A study was performed by the Obesity Society, stating that if you have your dinner before 2:00 p.m., your hunger yearnings will be reduced for the remainder of the day. At the same time, your fat-burning reserves are boosted. During the fasting period, you should only consume food items that have zero calories, including black coffee (a splash of cream is excellent), water, diet soda, and sugar-free gum.

Avoid These Food Items

- *Processed Meats:* While protein is an undeniably important part of a healthy diet, seeking your protein from meats, which have been treated, will overload your body full of chemicals. The processed meats tend to be lower in protein while higher in sodium and contain preservatives that can cause a variety of health risks, including asthma and heart disease. Choose from the quality cuts of meat found in most grocery stores.

- *White Flour:* Much like processed meats, by the time white flour has completed the processing, it's utterly devoid of any nutritional value. According to *Care2*, white flour, when consumed as part of a regular diet, has been shown to increase a woman's chance of breast cancer by a shocking 200%.

- *Non-Organic Milk:* Despite being touted as part of a balanced diet, non-organic milk is routinely found to be full of growth hormones. The growth hormones leave behind antibiotics, which, in turn, makes it more difficult for the human body to counter infections, causing an increased chance of colon cancer, prostate cancer, and breast cancer.

- *Farm-Raised Salmon:* Much like processed meat, farm-raised salmons are the least healthy type of an otherwise healthy meal choice. When salmons are raised in close proximity to one another for a prolonged period, they lose much of their natural vitamin D while picking up traces of PCB, DDT, carcinogens, and bromine.

- *Non-Organic Potatoes:* While the starch and carbohydrates it contains are a vital part of a balanced meal, non-organic potatoes are not worth the trouble. They are treated with chemicals while still in the ground, before being treated again; they are sent to the store as "fresh" as possible. These chemicals have been shown to increase the risk of things like birth defects, autism, asthma, learning disabilities, Parkinson's, and Alzheimer's disease, as well as multiple types of cancer.

Now that you have a good idea of how to proceed with your new way of eating, it is time to review all of the recipes.

Chapter 27:

Breakfast Favorites

Almond Coconut Egg Wraps

Serving Yields Provided: 4
Macro Counts - Each Serving:
- Net Carbs: 3 g
- Total Fats: 8 g
- Protein: 8 g
- Calories: 111

Ingredients Needed:
- Organic eggs (5)
- Almond meal (2 tbsp.)
- Sea salt (.25 tsp.)
- Coconut flour (1 tbsp.)

Directions for Preparation:
1. Combine the fixings in a blender and work until creamy.
2. Warm up a skillet using the medium-high temperature setting.
3. Pour 2 tbsp of batter into the pan and cover with a top.
4. Simmer for about 3 minutes.
5. Flip it over and continue cooking for an additional 3 minutes.
6. Serve hot.

Almonds & Chips Breakfast Cereal

Serving Yields Provided: 1
Macro Counts - Each Serving:
- Net Carbs: 3 g
- Protein: 6 g
- Total Fats: 27 g
- Calories: 300

Ingredients Needed:
- Coconut milk (.25 cup)
- Hemp hearts (3 tbsp.)
- Shredded coconut (.5 tbsp.)
- Chocolate chips (.5 tbsp.)
- Chopped almonds (.5 tbsp.)
- Liquid stevia (1 drop)

Directions for Preparation:
1. Store in the refrigerator for at least 4 hrs. Overnight is best.
2. Enjoy cold or warm.

Almost McGriddle Casserole

Serving Yields Provided: 8
Macro Counts - Each Serving:
- Net Carbs: 3 g
- Total Fats: 36 g
- Protein: 26 g
- Calories: 448

Ingredients Needed:
- Breakfast sausage (1 lb.)
- Flaxseed meal (.25 cup)
- Almond flour (1 cup)
- Large eggs (10)
- Maple syrup (6 tbsp.)
- Cheese (4 oz.)
- Butter (4 tbsp.)
- Onion (.5 tsp.)
- Sage (.25 tsp.)
- Garlic powder (.5 tsp.)
- *Also Needed*: 9 x 9-inch casserole dish & parchment baking paper

Directions for Preparation:
1. Heat the oven temperature to 350° Fahrenheit.

2. Use the medium heat setting on the stovetop to prepare the sausage in a skillet.
3. Add all of the dry ingredients (the cheese also), and stir in the wet ones. Add 4 tablespoons of the syrup. Stir and blend well.
4. After the sausage has browned, combine all of the fixings, along with the grease.
5. Prepare the casserole dish with a layer of baking paper. Empty the mix into the casserole dish and drizzle the rest of the syrup.
6. Bake for 45–55 minutes.
7. Transfer to the countertop and let it become room temperature. The casserole should be easy to remove by using the edge of the parchment paper.

Bacon Hash

Serving Yields Provided: 2
Macro Counts - Each Serving:
- Net Carbs: 9 g
- Total Fats: 24 g
- Protein: 23 g
- Calories: 366

Ingredients Needed:
- Bacon slices (6)
- Small onion (1)
- Small green pepper (1)
- Jalapenos (2)
- Eggs (4)

Directions for Preparation:
1. Chop the bacon into chunks using a food processor. Set aside for now.
2. Slice the peppers and onions into thin strips, and dice the jalapenos as small as possible.
3. Prepare a skillet with a spritz of non-stick cooking oil spray and fry the veggies.

4. Once browned, combine all of the fixings and cook until crispy.
5. Place on a serving dish with the eggs.

Bagels & Cheese

Serving Yields Provided: 6
Macro Counts - Each Serving:
- Net Carbs: 8 g
- Total Fats: 31 g
- Protein: 19 g
- Calories: 374

Ingredients Needed:
- Cream cheese (3 oz.)
- Baking powder (1 tsp.)
- Shredded mozzarella cheese (2.5 cups)
- Almond flour (1.5 cups)
- Eggs (2)

Directions for Preparation:
1. Combine the baking powder, mozzarella, flour, and cream cheese in a mixing container. Place in the microwave to melt for about 1 minute. Stir well.
2. Let the mixture cool and add the eggs. Break apart into six sections and shape into round bagels.
3. *Note*: You can also sprinkle with a seasoning of your choice or pinch of salt if desired.
4. Bake until the edges of the bagels are golden brown (12 to 15 min.).
5. Cool and store.

Belgian Style Waffles

Serving Yields Provided: 4
Macro Counts - Each Serving:
- Net Carbs: 3 g
- Total Fats: 19g
- Protein: 11 g
- Calories: 247

Ingredients Needed:
- Melted butter or ghee (4 tbsp.)
- Eggs (6)
- Salt (.5 tsp.)
- Bak. powder (.5 tsp.)
- Coconut flour (.33 cup)
- *Optional:* Sweet Leaf stevia drops (.125 tsp.)

Directions for Preparation:
1. In a blender, mix the butter and eggs until incorporated.
2. Pour in the salt, stevia, and baking powder. Blend well to combine.
3. Fold in the flour, and let it rest to thicken (5 min.)
4. Pour in small amounts of water as needed to thin the batter.
5. Prepare in the waffle maker and serve.

Biscuits & Gravy

Serving Yields Provided: 2
Macro Counts - Each Serving:
- Net Carbs: 2 g
- Total Fats: 36 g
- Protein: 22 g
- Calories: 425

Ingredients Needed:
- Salt (.25 tsp.)
- Almond flour (.25 cup)
- Baking powder (.5 tsp.)
- Large egg white (1)
- Crumbled breakfast sausage (6 oz.)
- Chicken broth (.25 cup)
- Cream cheese (.25 cup)
- Pepper & Salt (to your liking)

Directions for Preparation:
1. Warm up the oven to 400° Fahrenheit.
2. Prepare a baking tin with parchment baking paper.
3. Whisk the salt, almond flour, and baking powder.
4. In another dish, whisk the egg whites to form stiff peaks.
5. Dice the butter into small bits. Form a crumbled mixture in the dry components using the butter. Gently blend it into the egg whites.
6. Split the mixture of batter into two portions on the paper-lined pan. Bake for 11 to 15 minutes.
7. Using the medium heat setting, warm the sausage. When browned, add the cream cheese and chicken broth. Simmer and dust with pepper and salt.
8. Serve with the piping hot biscuits with a serving of the delicious gravy.

Blueberry Flaxseed Muffins

Serving Yields Provided: 10
Macro Counts - Each Serving:
- Net Carbs: 8.78 g
- Total Fats: 18.3g
- Protein: 7.57 g
- Calories: 221

Ingredients Needed:
- Flaxseeds (1.5 cups)
- Baking powder (1 tbsp.)
- Eggs (5)
- Vanilla extract (1 tsp.)
- Almond milk (3 tbsp.)
- Coconut oil (4 tbsp.)
- Blueberries (.5 cup)
- Salt (1 pinch)
- Sugar substitute (to your liking)

Directions for Preparation:
1. Warm up the oven to reach 350° Fahrenheit.
2. Use a coffee grinder to prepare the seeds.
3. Combine each of the dry fixings in a mixing container.
4. Whisk the eggs in a mixing container. Pour in the oil and milk. Stir well.

5. Combine all of the fixings.
6. Fold in the berries and stir gently with a spoon.
7. Pour into muffin cups.
8. Bake for 15 minutes. Cool slightly and serve.

Blueberry Ricotta Pancakes

Serving Yields Provided: 5
Macro Counts - Each Serving:
- Net Carbs: 6 g
- Total Fats: 23 g
- Protein: 15 g
- Calories: 311

Ingredients Needed:
- Ricotta (.75 cup)
- Large eggs (3)
- Unsweetened vanilla almond milk (.25 cup)
- Golden flaxseed meal (.5 cup)
- Salt (.25 tsp.)
- Baking powder (1 tsp.)
- Almond flour (1 cup)
- Stevia powder (.5 tsp.)
- Vanilla extract (.5 tsp.)
- Blueberries (.25 cup)
- *Optional*: Keto-friendly syrup of choice; add the carbs

Directions for Preparation:
1. Blend the eggs, milk, ricotta, and vanilla extract with an electric mixer.
2. Combine the flaxseed meal, salt, flour, baking powder, and stevia in another dish.
3. Add the dry ingredients into the blender—slowly—to form the batter. Use two to three blueberries for each pancake.
4. Add the butter to a preheated skillet using a medium heat setting. When it melts, add the batter using two tablespoons for each scoop.
5. At this point, serve or set aside to cool.

6. You can serve or freeze to use later if you have limited time. If you know your schedule will be rushed, you can pour the syrup in a cup with a lid.
7. Enjoy with a side of bacon, but add the additional carbs to the count.

Chocolate Loaf

Serving Yields Provided: 8
Macro Counts - Each Serving:
- Net Carbs: 2.32 g
- Total Fats: 17.8g
- Protein: 5.7 g
- Calories: 195

Ingredients Needed:
- Large eggs (6)
- Coconut flour (.75 cup)
- Butter (4 oz.)
- Unsweetened cocoa powder (.33 cup)
- Bak. soda (.5 tsp.)
- Salt (1 pinch)
- Bak. powder (1 tsp.)
- Sugar substitute (as desired)
- Apple cider vinegar (2 tsp.)
- *Also Needed*: Parchment paper

Directions for Preparation:
1. Warm the oven to reach 350° Fahrenheit.
2. Line the baking pan with the paper.
3. Whisk the eggs and stir in the melted butter.
4. Sift the dry fixings. Pour in the wet mixture, and add the vinegar.
5. Stir well and pour into the pan.
6. Bake for 20 to 30 minutes.
7. Serve after testing its doneness (if the toothpick inserted in the center comes out clean.

Cinnamon Raisin Bagels

Serving Yields Provided: 6
Macro Counts - Each Serving:
- Net Carbs: 6 g
- Total Fats: 10 g
- Protein: 3 g
- Calories: 139

Ingredients Needed:
- Coconut flour sifted (.33 cup)
- Golden flax meal (1.5 tbsp.)
- Baking soda (.5 tsp.)
- *Optional:* Sea salt (a dash)
- Baking powder (1 tsp.)
- Cinnamon (2 tsp.)
- Whisked eggs (3)
- Apple cider vinegar (1 tsp.)
- Unsweetened coconut or almond milk (.33 cup)
- Melted butter - coconut oil or ghee (2.5 tbsp.)
- Liquid stevia (1 tsp.)
- Golden raisins (.33 cup)
- *Optional*: Vanilla extract (1 tsp.)
- *Also Needed:* Donut/bagel pan

Directions for Preparation:
1. Warm up the oven to 350° Fahrenheit.
2. Grease the pan.
3. Mix the dry fixings (the golden flax meal, the sifted coconut flour, baking soda, cinnamon, sea salt, and baking powder) thoroughly.
4. In another container, combine the almond/coconut milk, apple cider vinegar, eggs, melted butter/coconut oil, vanilla extract, and stevia.
5. Combine all of the fixings and add to the prepared pan, spreading evenly with a spatula.
6. Bake for 17 to 20 minutes. Cool for 3 to 4 minutes.
7. Loosen the bagels with a knife. Turn the bread on the side and slice into half.
8. Serve with toppings of your choice, such as butter or cream cheese.
9. Refrigerate or freeze unused portions.

Classic Bacon & Eggs

Serving Yields Provided:
Macro Counts - Each Serving:
- Net Carbs: 1 g
- Total Fats: 22 g
- Protein: 15g
- Calories: 272

Ingredients Needed:
- Eggs (8)
- Sliced bacon (5 oz.)
- *Optional:* Cherry tomatoes & Fresh parsley

Directions for Preparation:
1. Prepare the bacon in a skillet using the medium-high temperature until crispy. Leave the rendered fat in the pan, and put the bacon in a platter to drain.
2. Fry the eggs in the bacon remnants using medium heat.
3. Cook the eggs any way you like them. For a *Sunny Side Up*, leave the eggs to fry on one side. Cover the pan with a lid to make sure they get cooked on top. For *Over-Easy Eggs*, flip the eggs over after a few minutes and cook for another minute.
4. Slice the cherry tomatoes in half, and fry them at the same time.
5. Dust with pepper and salt to your liking.

Cocoa Waffles

Serving Yields Provided: 5
Macro Counts - Each Serving:
- Net Carbs: 3.4 g
- Protein: 7 g
- Total Fats: 27 g
- Calories: 289

Ingredients Needed:
- Separated eggs (5)
- Unsweetened cocoa (.25 cup)
- Granular sweetener (3 tbsp.)
- Coconut flour (4 tbsp.)
- Baking powder (1 tsp.)
- Melted butter (4.5 oz.)
- Milk of choice (3 tbsp.)
- Vanilla (1 tsp.)

Directions for Preparation:
1. Use a whisk to prepare the egg whites. Briskly mix to form stiff peaks.
2. In another container, whisk the sweetener, baking powder, and cocoa with the egg yolks.
3. Add the butter to the dry mixture. Stir in the vanilla and milk.
4. Fold in the prepared egg whites, a little at a time.
5. Transfer the mixture in the waffle maker.
6. Cook until they are golden brown.
7. Serve.

Corned Beef & Radish Hash

Serving Yields Provided: 4
Macro Counts - Each Serving - 0.5 cup each:
- Net Carbs: 1.5 g
- Total Fats: 16 g
- Protein: 23 g
- Calories: 252

Ingredients Needed:
- Olive oil (1 tbsp.)
- Diced onions (.25 cup)
- Radishes (1 cup)
- Kosher salt (.5 tsp.)
- Garlic powder (.25 tsp.)
- Black pepper (.25 tsp.)
- Dried oregano (.5 tsp.)
- Corned beef (12 oz. can) or Finely chopped, packed corned beef (1 cup)

Directions for Preparation:
1. Dice the radishes to .5-inch cuts.
2. Warm the oil in a large sauté pan. Toss in the onions, radishes, salt, and pepper.
3. Sauté the onions and radishes on medium heat until softened (5 min.).
4. Add the oregano, garlic powder, and corned beef to the pan and stir well until combined.
5. Cook using low to medium heat, occasionally stirring for 10 minutes or until the radishes are soft and starting to brown.
6. Press the mixture into the bottom of the pan and cook on high heat for 2 to 3 minutes or until the bottom is crisp and brown.
7. Serve hot.

Creamy Basil Baked Sausage

Serving Yields Provided: 12
Macro Counts - Each Serving:
- Net Carbs: 4 g
- Total Fats: 23 g
- Protein: 23 g
- Calories: 316

Ingredients Needed:
- Italian sausage, pork, turkey, or chicken (3 lb.)
- Cream cheese (8 oz.)
- Heavy cream (.25 cup)
- Basil pesto (.25 cup)
- Mozzarella (8 oz.)

Directions for Preparation:

1. Warm up the oven to reach 400° Fahrenheit.
2. Lightly spritz a casserole dish with cooking oil spray. Add the sausage to the dish and bake for 30 minutes.
3. Combine the heavy cream, pesto, and cream cheese.
4. Once the sauce is done, pour it over the casserole. Top it off with the cheese.
5. Bake for another 10 minutes. The sausage should reach 160° Fahrenheit in the center when checked with a meat thermometer.
6. *Option 2*: You can also broil for 3 minutes to brown the cheesy layer.

Eggs & Sausage Breakfast Sandwich

Serving Yields Provided: 1
Macro Counts - Each Serving:
- Net Carbs: 6 g
- Protein: 32g
- Total Fats: 8 g
- Calories: 880

Ingredients Needed:
- Butter (1 tbsp.)
- Large eggs (2)
- Mayonnaise (1 tbsp.)
- Sausage patties, cooked (2)
- Sharp cheddar cheese (2 slices)
- Avocado (2-3 slices)

Directions for Preparation:

1. Warm and melt the butter in a large skillet using the medium heat setting. Place lightly oiled Mason jar rings or silicone egg molds into the pan.
2. Crack the eggs into the rings and use a fork to break the yolks. Gently whisk.
3. Place a lid on the pot and cook for 3 to 4 minutes or until eggs are cooked

through. Remove the eggs from the rings.

4. Place one of the eggs on a plate and top it with half of the mayonnaise. Top the eggs with one of the sausage patties, a slice of cheese, and the avocado.
5. Put the second sausage patty on top of the avocado, and top it with the remaining cheese. Spread the remaining mayonnaise on the second cooked egg, and put it on top of the cheese. Serve.

Green Buttered Eggs

Serving Yields Provided: 2
Macro Counts - Each Serving:
- Net Carbs: 2.5 g
- Total Fats: 27.5 g
- Protein: 12.8 g
- Calories: 311

Ingredients Needed:
- Coconut oil (1 tbsp.)
- Organic butter (2 tbsp.)
- Cloves of garlic (2)
- Fresh cilantro (.5 cup)
- Fresh parsley (.5 cup)
- Fresh thyme leaves (1 tsp.)
- Organic eggs (4)
- Ground cayenne (.25 tsp.)
- Sea salt (.25 tsp.)
- Ground cumin (.25 tsp.)

Directions for Preparation:

1. Mince the garlic, and finely chop the parsley and cilantro.
2. Heat a skillet, melting the oil and butter. Toss in the garlic and sauté about 3 minutes (low setting). Add the thyme. Sauté for another 30 seconds.
3. Toss in the cilantro and parsley using the medium heat setting about three more minutes.

4. Break in the eggs (don't break the yolk).
5. Cover and cook about four to 6 minutes until the yolks are set (runny yolk cooks in 3 to 4 minutes).
6. Serve right away and enjoy.

Keto Hot Cross Buns

Serving Yields Provided: 8
Macro Counts - Each Serving:
- Net Carbs: 2.1 g
- Total Fats: 3.1 g
- Protein: 5.6 g
- Calories: 84

Ingredients Needed:
- Coconut flour (.33 cup)
- Psyllium husks (.33 cup)
- Baking powder (1 tsp.)
- Swerve granulated sweetener (2 tbsp. or more to taste)
- Salt (.5 tsp.)
- Pumpkin spice (.5 tsp.)
- Cinnamon (.5 tsp.)
- Ground cloves (.5 tsp.)
- Eggs (4 medium)
- Boiling water (1 cup
- Raisins/cacao nibs/chocolate chips
- Powdered sweetener icing mix

Directions for Preparation:
1. Mix each of the dry fixings in a mixing bowl.
2. Whisk and fold in the eggs.
3. Pour in the boiling water and mix until evenly combined.
4. Roll into eight equal balls. Add to a baking pan.
5. Bake in a fan-assisted oven at 350° Fahrenheit for 20–30 minutes.
6. Make the icing. Mark each hot cross bun with a cross using a keto-friendly powdered sweetener confectioners/icing mix and water paste mixture.

Lavender Biscuits

Serving Yields Provided: 6
Macro Counts - Each Serving:
- Net Carbs: 4 g
- Total Fats: 25 g
- Protein: 10 g
- Calories: 270

Ingredients Needed:
- Coconut oil (.33 cup)
- Almond flour (1.5 cups)
- Egg whites (4)
- Kosher salt (1 pinch)
- Baking powder (1 tsp.)
- Culinary grade lavender buds (1 tbsp.)
- Liquid stevia (4 drops)

Directions for Preparation:
1. Warm up the oven until it reaches 350° Fahrenheit.
2. Spritz a baking sheet with a little coconut oil.
3. Combine the almond flour and coconut oil in a mixing container until it's pea-sized pieces. Set the bowl aside in the fridge.
4. Whisk the eggs until they start foaming. Toss in the salt, lavender, and baking powder. Stir well and mix in the eggs. Mix in with the almond mixture, stirring well.
5. Place the biscuits onto the baking sheet using an ice cream scoop or tablespoon. Pat them, so they become round like a pancake.
6. Bake for 20 minutes and serve.

Pesto Scrambled Eggs

Serving Yields Provided: 1
Macro Counts - Each Serving:
- Net Carbs: 2.6 g
- Total Fats: 41.5 g
- Protein: 20.4 g
- Calories: 467

Ingredients Needed:
- Eggs (3 large)
- Pesto, green or red (1 tbsp.)
- Butter/Ghee (1 tbsp.)
- Creamed coconut milk/soured cream/crème Fraiche (2 tbsp.)
- Freshly ground black pepper & Himalayan salt (as desired)

Directions for Preparation:
1. Whisk the eggs. Sprinkle with pepper and salt to your liking.
2. Prepare a pan with the butter and wait for it to melt.
3. Combine and prepare the fixings using the low heat setting. Stir well and add the pesto.
4. Take the skillet off of the burner and blend in the crème Fraiche.
5. Combine well. Serve any way you choose.

Porridge

Serving Yields Provided: 1
Macro Counts - Each Serving:
- Net Carbs: 5.4 g
- Total Fats: 22.8 g
- Protein: 10.1 g
- Calories: 401

Ingredients Needed:
- Salt (1 pinch)
- Coconut cream (4 tbsp.)
- Psyllium husk powder (1 pinch ground)
- Coconut flour (1 tbsp.)
- Flaxseed Egg (1)
- Coconut butter (1 oz.)

Directions for Preparation:
1. Add all of the fixings into a pan, and place it on the stovetop using the low heat setting.
2. Stir continuously to encourage the porridge to thicken. Continue stirring until your preferred thickness is reached.

3. A small amount of coconut milk or a few berries (fresh or frozen) can also be added, to taste.

Pulled Pork Hash

Serving Yields Provided: 2
Macro Counts - Each Serving:
- Net Carbs: 8 g
- Total Fats: 22 g
- Protein: 21 g
- Calories: 354

Ingredients Needed:
- Lard or fat of choice (2 tbsp.)
- Turnip (1)
- Paprika (.5 tsp.)
- Garlic powder (.25 tsp.)
- Black pepper & salt (.25 tsp. each)
- Brussels sprouts (3)
- Lacinato kale (about 2 leaves, 1 cup)
- Red onion (2 tbsp.)
- Pulled pork (3 oz.)
- Eggs (2)
- *Also Needed*: Large cast-iron skillet

Directions for Preparation:
1. Dice the turnip and slice the Brussel sprouts into halves. Chop the kale and dice the onion.
2. Warm up the oil in a skillet using a medium-high temperature setting. Add the diced turnip and the spices.
3. Cook for approximately 5 minutes.
4. Stir in the rest of the vegetables and cook for another two to 3 minutes until they start to soften.
5. Add in the pork and cook for two more minutes.
6. Make two divots in the hash and crack in the eggs.
7. Cover and cook for 3 to 5 minutes just until the whites are set.

Pumpkin Pancakes

Serving Yields Provided: 1
Macro Counts - Each Serving:
- Net Carbs: 4 g
- Total Fats: 56 g
- Protein: 9 g
- Calories: 551

Ingredients Needed:
- Coconut oil (2 tbsp.)
- Eggs (2)
- Cinnamon (.25 tsp.)
- Vanilla extract (.25 tsp.)
- Pumpkin puree (.25 cup)
- Coconut flour (2 tbsp.)
- Butter (2 tbsp.)

Directions for Preparation:
1. Whisk the eggs and puree with the cinnamon and vanilla extract.
2. Slowly, add the coconut flour, whisking until the lumps are gone.
3. Warm up the oil using the medium heat setting.
4. Once the pan is hot, prepare the pancakes until it starts to bubble.
5. Turn it over. Cook until golden brown. Serve with the butter.

Sage & Sausage Patties

Serving Yields Provided: 8
Macro Counts - Each Serving:
- Net Carbs: 1.4 g
- Total Fats: 11 g
- Protein: 21 g - Calories: 187

Ingredients Needed:
- Maple extract (1 tsp.)
- Granular swerve sweetener (2 tbsp.)
- Garlic powder (.25 tsp.)
- Pepper (.5 tsp.)
- Cayenne (.125 tsp.)
- Salt (1 tsp.)
- Freshly chopped sage (2 tbsp.)
- Ground pork (1 lb.)
- *For the Pan*: Olive oil (1 tsp.)

Directions for Preparation:
1. Whisk each of the fixings in a mixing container and add the pork. Mix well.
2. Shape the patties to approximately a 1-inch thickness.
3. Add the olive oil or some of the butter to a pan on the stovetop using the medium heat setting. Cook each side for 3 to 4 minutes.

Smoothie in a Bowl

Serving Yields Provided: 1
Macro Counts - Each Serving:
- Net Carbs: 4 g
- Total Fats: 35 g
- Protein: 35 g
- Calories: 570

Ingredients Needed:
- Almond milk (.5 cup)
- Spinach (1 cup)
- Heavy cream (2 tbsp.)
- Low-carb protein powder (1 scoop)
- Coconut oil (1 tbsp.)
- Ice (2 cubes)

Ingredients Needed - The Toppings:
- Walnuts (4)
- Raspberries (4)
- Chia seeds 1 tsp.)
- Shredded coconut (1 tbsp.)

Directions for Preparation:
1. Add a cup of spinach to your high-speed blender. Pour in the cream, almond milk, ice, and coconut oil.
2. Blend for a few seconds until it has an even consistency, and all ingredients are combined well. Empty the goodies into a serving dish.
3. Arrange your toppings or give them a toss and mix them together. Of course, you can make it pretty by alternating the strips of toppings.

Spinach Quiche

Serving Yields Provided: 6
Macro Counts - Each Serving:
- Net Carbs: 0 g
- Total Fats: 23 g
- Protein: 19g
- Calories: 299

Ingredients Needed:
- Chopped onion (1)
- Olive oil (1 tbsp.)
- Frozen & thawed spinach (10 oz. pkg.)
- Shredded Muenster cheese (3 cups)
- Organic eggs, whisked (5)
- *To Taste*: Black pepper and salt
- *Also Needed*: 9-inch pie plate

Directions for Preparation:
1. Warm the oven in advance to reach 350° Fahrenheit. Lightly grease the dish.
2. Use the medium heat setting to warm a skillet with the oil.
3. Toss in the onions and saute for 4 to 5 minutes. Raise the heat setting to medium-high.
4. Fold in the spinach. Sauté for about two to 3 minutes or until the liquid is absorbed. Cool slightly.
5. Combine the rest of the fixings in a large mixing container and toss with the cooled spinach. Dump into the prepared dish and bake for 30 minutes.
6. Take the quiche out of the oven and cool for at least 10 minutes.
7. Slice into six wedges.

Tomato Pesto Mug Cake

Serving Yields Provided: 1
Macro Counts - Each Serving:
- Net Carbs: 4 g
- Total Fats: 45 g
- Protein: 13 g
- Calories: 460

Ingredients Needed:
- Large egg (1)
- Almond flour (2 tbsp.)
- Butter (2 tbsp.)
- Baking powder (.5 tsp.)

Ingredients Needed - The Pesto:
- Almond flour (1 tbsp.)
- Sun-dried tomato pesto (5 tsp.)
- Salt (1 pinch)

Directions for Preparation:
1. Combine each of the fixings in a mug, but keep a little pesto for the garnish.
2. Microwave the cup for 70–80 seconds.
3. Lightly tap the mug on a serving dish. It will fall right out.
4. Top the cake with the pesto and serve.

Chapter 28:

Lunchtime Options

Bread Twists for the Salad

Serving Yields Provided: 10
Macro Counts - Each Serving:
- Net Carbs: 1 g
- Total Fats: 18 g
- Protein: 7 g
- Calories: 204

Ingredients Needed:
- Almond flour (.5 cup)
- Coconut flour (4 tbsp.)
- Salt (.5 tsp.)
- Baking powder (1 tsp.)
- Shredded cheese, your choice (1.5 cups)
- Butter (2.33 oz.)
- Egg (2, use 1 for brushing the tops)
- Green pesto (2 oz.)

Directions for Preparation:
1. Warm up the oven to reach 350° Fahrenheit. Prepare a cookie sheet with a layer of parchment paper.
2. Mix all of the dry fixings.
3. Use the low heat setting to melt the butter and cheese together. Stir until smooth and add the egg. Stir well.
4. Combine all of the fixings to make the dough.
5. Roll out the dough between the two layers of parchment paper until it is about 1-inch thick. Remove the top sheet.
6. Spread the pesto on top of the dough and slice into 1-inch strips.
7. Twist the dough and arrange on the baking tin. Brush the twists with the second egg (gently whisked).
8. Bake until golden brown, about 15 to 20 minutes.

Caprese Salad

Serving Yields Provided: 4
Macro Counts - Each Serving:
- Net Carbs: 4.6 g
- Total Fats: 63.5 g
- Protein: 7.7 g
- Calories: 191

Ingredients Needed:
- Grape tomatoes (3 cups)
- Peeled garlic cloves (4)
- Avocado oil (2 tbsp.)
- Mozzarella balls (10 pearl-sized)
- Baby spinach leaves (4 cups)
- Fresh basil leaves (.25 cup)
- Brine reserved from the cheese (1 tbsp.)
- Pesto (1 tbsp.)

Directions for Preparation:
1. Program the oven setting to 400° Fahrenheit.
2. Prepare a baking tin with a layer of aluminum foil.
3. Arrange the tomatoes and cloves in the prepared pan. Spritz with the oil. Bake 20-30 minutes or until the tops are slightly browned.
4. Drain the liquid (saving 1 tbsp) from the brine. Mix the pesto with the brine.

5. Arrange the spinach in a large salad container. Transfer the tomatoes to the dish, along with the roasted garlic. Drizzle with the pesto sauce.
6. Garnish with the mozzarella balls and freshly torn basil leaves.

Chicken BLT Salad

Serving Yields Provided: 4
Macro Counts - Each Serving:
- Net Carbs: 4 g
- Total Fats: 78g
- Protein: 28 g
- Calories: 837

Ingredients Needed:
- Boneless chicken thighs (1 lb.)
- Butter (1 oz.)
- Bacon (.5 lb.)
- Cherry tomatoes (4 oz.)
- Romaine lettuce (10 oz.)
- Salt and pepper (to your liking)

Ingredients Needed - Garlic Mayonnaise:
- Mayonnaise (.75 cup)
- Garlic powder (.5 tbsp.)

Directions for Preparation:
1. Whisk the mayonnaise and garlic powder in a small bowl and set aside for now.
2. Fry the bacon in butter until crispy. Transfer to a dish to drain and keep warm. Save the grease in the pan.
3. Shred the chicken and dust using the salt and pepper. Fry in the same skillet as the bacon until golden brown.
4. Rinse and shred the lettuce.
5. Toss the lettuce on a plate and top with chicken, bacon, tomatoes, and a serving of garlic mayonnaise.

Chicken, Feta, & Kiwi Salad

Serving Yields Provided: 2
Macro Counts - Each Serving:
- Net Carbs: 13 g
- Total Fats: 15 g
- Protein: 28 g
- Calories: 314

Ingredients Needed:
- Fig balsamic vinegar (1 tbsp.)
- Kiwis (2)
- Extra-virgin olive oil (1 tbsp.)
- Salt (1 pinch)
- Mixed field greens (4 cups)
- Chopped grilled chicken breast (1 cup, about 5 oz.)
- Feta cheese (.33 cup)

Directions for Preparation:
1. Chop the chicken and crumble the feta.
2. Whisk the balsamic vinegar, oil, and salt.
3. Add the greens and chicken breast.
4. Peel and cut the kiwi into halves. Dice into 1-inch wedges and add to the salad with the crumbled feta.
5. Toss well to combine.

Chicken-Pecan Salad & Cucumber Bites

Serving Yields Provided: 2
Macro Counts - Each Serving:
- Net Carbs: 3 g
- Total Fats: 24 g
- Protein: 23 g
- Calories: 323

Ingredients Needed:
- Mayonnaise (2 tbsp.)
- Precooked chicken breast (1 cup)
- Cucumber (1)
- Diced celery (.25 cup)
- Chopped pecans (.25 cup)

- Pink salt—Himalayan & Black pepper (1 pinch of each)

Directions for Preparation:
1. Peel and slice the cucumber into 1/4-inch slices. Dice the chicken and celery. Chop the pecans.
2. Combine the pecans, chicken, mayo, and celery in a salad bowl. Sprinkle with pepper and salt.
3. Lay the cucumber slices on a platter, and add a pinch of salt. Layer each one with a spoonful of the chicken salad. Serve.

Cobb Salad

Serving Yields Provided: 2
Macro Counts - Each Serving:
- Net Carbs: 3 g
- Total Fats: 48 g
- Protein: 43 g
- Calories: 600

Ingredients Needed:
- Hard-boiled egg (1)
- Spinach (1 cup)
- Bacon strips (2)
- Campari tomato (.5 of 1)
- Chicken breast (2 oz.)
- Avocado (.25 of 1)
- Olive oil (1 tbsp.)
- White vinegar (.5 tsp.)

Directions for Preparation:
1. Prepare the bacon and chicken shred or slice the chicken.
2. Cut all of the ingredients into small pieces.
3. Toss them to a bowl with the vinegar and oil. Toss gently and serve.

Egg Salad

Serving Yields Provided: 4
Macro Counts - Each Serving:
- Net Carbs: 1.4 g
- Total Fats: 29 g

- Protein: 8.7 g
- Calories: 305

Ingredients Needed:
- Hard-boiled eggs (6)
- Curry Powder (1 tsp. or to taste)
- Full-fat Mayonnaise (.5 cup)

Directions for Preparation:
1. Prepare the boiled eggs by adding them into a saucepan. Pour in *cold* water.
2. Turn the burner on.
3. Once the water begins to boil, set a timer for 7 minutes and then pour the hot water when done.
4. Prepare a cold-water bath, and submerge the hot eggs into it to stop the cooking process.
5. When cooled, peel and chop the eggs into small bits.
6. Combine the mayo, eggs, and curry powder.
7. Serve with a portion of chopped fresh parsley.

Greek Salad

Serving Yields Provided: 1
Macro Counts - Each Serving:
- Net Carbs: 8 g
- Total Fats: 57.5 g
- Protein: 12 g
- Calories: 594

Ingredients Needed:
- Red onion (.25 cup)
- Tomato (.25 cup)
- Olive oil (3 tbsp.)
- Cucumber (.25 cup)
- Bell pepper (.25 cup)
- Feta cheese (.5 cup)
- Olives (1 tbsp.)
- Red wine vinegar (.5 tbsp.)

Directions for Preparation:

1. Dice the tomato, chop the olives, and slice the onion, cucumber, and pepper. Combine the bell pepper with the tomato, cucumber, crumbled feta cheese, and onion.
2. Spritz using the oil and vinegar with a shake of pepper and salt to your liking.
3. Toss until all of the ingredients are mixed well before serving.

Healthy Thai Pork Salad

Serving Yields Provided: 2
Macro Counts - Each Serving:
- Net Carbs: 5.2 g
- Total Fats: 33 g
- Protein: 29 g
- Calories: 461

Ingredients Needed - The Sauce:
- Juice & zest of lime (1 lime)
- Chopped cilantro (2 tbsp.)
- Tomato paste (2 tbsp.)
- Soy sauce (2 tbsp. + 2 tsp.)
- Red curry paste (1 tsp.)
- Five Spice (1 tsp.)
- Fish sauce (1 tsp.)
- Red pepper flakes (.25 tsp.)
- Rice wine vinegar (1 tbsp. + 1 tsp.)
- Mango extract (.5 tsp.)
- Liquid stevia (10 drops)

Ingredients Needed - The Salad:
- Romaine lettuce (2 cups)
- Pulled pork (10 oz.)
- Medium chopped red bell pepper (.25 of 1)
- Chopped cilantro (.25 cup)

Directions for Preparation:
1. Zest half of the lime, and chop the cilantro.
2. Mix all of the sauce fixings.
3. Blend the barbecue sauce components and set aside.

4. Pull the pork apart, and make the salad. Pour glaze over the pork with a bit of the sauce.

Jalapeno Popper Chicken Salad

Serving Yields Provided: 4
Macro Counts - Each Serving:
- Net Carbs: 0 g - Total Fats: 38.7 g
- Protein: 46.6 g
- Calories: 532

Ingredients Needed:
- Chicken breast (1.5 lb.)
- Bacon (8 slices, 8 oz.)
- Jalapeños (3)
- Chopped green onion (.5 cup)
- Sour cream or dairy-free mayonnaise (.5 cup)
- Hot sauce (2 tbsp.)
- Garlic powder (.5 tsp.)
- Black pepper (.5 tsp.)
- Salt (.5 tsp.)

Directions for Preparation:
1. Warm the oven to reach 450° Fahrenheit.
2. Prepare a baking sheet with a layer of parchment baking paper.
3. Place raw chicken breast on top of the paper, and place the baking sheet to the oven. Cook until the internal temperature reaches 165° Fahrenheit or about 15 to 18 minutes. Transfer to a large platter and chill slightly.
4. Reduce the oven temperature setting to 425° Fahrenheit.
5. Bake the bacon in the oven until it's crispy (15-20 min.). Transfer to a paper towel-lined plated to remove excess grease. Set aside.
6. Turn on the oven broiler, and prepare a baking tin with paper. Put the jalapeños atop the paper and broil until lightly charred (3 min.).

Remove the jalapeños from the oven. Cool slightly before roughly chopping. De-seed jalapeños based on your spice preferences. Transfer the jalapeños to a large mixing bowl.

7. Remove the cooked chicken from the fridge and cube. Crumble the cooked bacon. Transfer both to the mixing bowl of chopped jalapeños.

8. Toss in the rest of the fixings and mix until well-combined.

9. Cover the bowl with a top or foil, and transfer it to the refrigerator to chill for 1 hour before serving.

Jar Salad With Tempeh – Vegan

Serving Yields Provided: 1
Macro Counts - Each Serving:
- Net Carbs: 4 g
- Protein: 8.1 g
- Total Fats: 18.7 g - Calories: 215

Ingredients Needed:
- Black pepper & salt (as desired)
- Keto-friendly mayonnaise (4 tbsp.)
- Scallion (.5)
- Cucumber (.25 oz.)
- Red bell pepper (.25 oz.)
- Cherry tomatoes (.25 oz.)
- Leafy greens (.25 oz.)
- Seasoned tempeh (4 oz.)

Directions for Preparation:
1. Chop or shred the vegetables as desired. Layer in the dark leafy greens first, followed by the onions, tomatoes, bell peppers, avocado, and shredded carrot.

2. Top the veggies off with the tempeh or use the same amount of another high-protein option to mix things up in later weeks.

3. Top with keto-vegan mayonnaise before serving.

Kale Salad

Serving Yields Provided: 4
Macro Counts - Each Serving:
- Net Carbs: 3 g
- Total Fats: 6 g
- Protein: 4 g
- Calories: 80

Ingredients Needed:
- Salt (.5 tsp.)
- Olive oil (1 tbsp.)
- Kale (1 bunch)
- Lemon juice (1 tbsp.)
- Parmesan cheese (.33 cup)

Directions for Preparation:
1. Use a sharp knife to discard the ribs from the kale and slice into ¼-inch strips.

2. Combine with the salt and oil and toss for about 3 minutes until softened.

3. Toss the cheese, juice, and kale. Serve.

Simple Red Cabbage Salad

Serving Yields Provided: 4
Macro Counts - Each Serving:
- Net Carbs: 0.2 g
- Protein: 3 g
- Total Fats: 3 g
- Calories: 131

Ingredients Needed:
- Shredded red cabbage (2 cups)
- Pepper and salt (as desired)
- Coconut sugar (.5 tsp.)
- Red wine vinegar (2 tsp.)
- Coconut oil (1 tbsp.)
- Chopped onion (.25 cup)

Directions for Preparation:
1. Place the steamer basket in the Kitchen robot and add the red cabbage.

2. Lock the top. Set the timer for 1 to 2 minutes. Quick-release the pressure, and remove the basket.
3. Rinse the cabbage under cold water and arrange in four portions.
4. Add the fixings, toss, and serve.

Tuna Salad & Chives

Serving Yields Provided: 4
Macro Counts - Each Serving:
- Net Carbs: 1 g
- Total Fats: 18 g
- Protein: 20 g
- Calories: 235

Ingredients Needed:
- Tuna in olive oil (15 oz.)
- Mayonnaise (6 tbsp.)
- Chives (2 tbsp.)
- Pepper (.25 tsp.)
- Salt (to taste)

Directions for Preparation:
1. Drain the tuna and finely chop the chives.
2. Add all of the fixings except the lettuce into a mixing bowl.
3. Toss well.
4. Enjoy as-is or spoon into romaine lettuce leaves.

Warm Peach Scallops Salad

Serving Yields Provided: 2
Macro Counts - Each Serving:
- Net Carbs: 7 g
- Total Fats: 8g
- Protein: 48 g
- Calories: 130

Ingredients Needed:
- Coconut oil, for the pan (as needed)
- Small scallops (12)
- Sliced peaches (1 whole)
- Sliced onion (.5 of 1)
- Oil (1 tsp.)
- Lemon juice (1 tsp.)
- Arugula leaves (5 oz.)

Directions for Preparation:
1. Warm up the oil in a skillet and add the scallops. Sauté for about 5 minutes per side.
2. Toss the arugula, onion slices, peaches, juice, and oil well.
3. When ready to serve, add the scallops on top of the mixture.

Vegetarian Club Salad

Serving Yields Provided: 3
Macro Counts - Each Serving:
- Net Carbs: 5 g
- Total Fats: 26 g
- Protein: 17 g
- Calories: 330

Ingredients Needed:
- Mayonnaise (2 tbsp.)
- Sour cream (2 tbsp.)
- Garlic powder (.5 tsp.)
- Dried parsley (1 tsp.)
- Onion powder (.5 tsp.)
- Milk (1 tbsp.)
- Dijon mustard (1 tbsp.)
- Large hard-boiled eggs (3)
- Cheddar cheese (4 oz.)
- Cherry tomatoes (.5 cup)
- Diced cucumber (1 cup)
- Torn romaine lettuce (3 cups)

Directions for Preparation:
1. Slice the hard-boiled eggs, and cube the cheese with a knife. Cut the tomatoes into halves, and dice the cucumber. Place the containers to the side for now.
2. Prepare the dressing (dried herbs, mayo, and sour cream) and mix well.
3. Add 1 tablespoon of milk to the mixture—and another if it's too thick.
4. Layer the salad with the vegetables, cheese, and egg slices. Scoop a

spoonful of mustard in the center, along with a drizzle of dressing.
5. Toss and enjoy!
6. *Notes:* The nutritional count is based on 2 tbsp of dressing.

Soup Choices

Broccoli Curry Soup

Serving Yields Provided: 4
Macro Counts - Each Serving:
- Net Carbs: 4.8 g
- Total Fats: 19.8 g
- Protein: 16.9 g
- Calories: 375

Ingredients Needed:
- Salt & Black pepper (as needed)
- Onion (1)
- Curry (1 tbsp.)
- Coconut oil (2 tbsp.)
- Vegetable stock (1 liter)
- Coconut cream (1 cup)
- Keto-friendly sharp cheese, your choice (.75 cup)
- Broccoli (1 lb.)

Directions for Preparation:
1. Pour the coconut oil into a frying pan on the stovetop over a burner turned to the medium-high heat setting.
2. Chop the onion and add to the pan. Simmer for approximately 6 minutes.
3. Lower the temperature to medium. Then, add in the broth until it begins to simmer. Mix in the broccoli, as well as any seasonings before adding in the curry and letting it simmer for 20 minutes.
4. Pour into a blender before mixing in the cheese substitute.
5. Blend well.

Chicken Chowder – Crockpot

Serving Yields Provided: 4
Macro Counts - Each Serving:
- Net Carbs: 7.5 g
- Total Fats: 28.8 g
- Protein: 40 g
- Calories: 457

Ingredients Needed:
- Garlic clove (1)
- Cilantro (1 tbsp.)
- Small onion (1)
- Cream cheese (8 oz.)
- Chicken broth (1 cup)
- Chicken breasts (1 lb.)
- Diced tomatoes (14 oz.)
- Diced jalapeno (.5 oz.)
- Fresh lime juice (1.6 oz.)
- Black pepper (1 tbsp.)
- Salt (1 tsp.)

Directions for Preparation:
1. Remove the skin and bones from the chicken.
2. Chop the garlic and cilantro. Dice the onion and jalapeno.
3. Combine all of the fixings in the crockpot.
4. Prepare using the low-temperature setting for 6 to 9 hours or high for 4 hours.
5. Once it is done, shred the chicken in the pot using two forks.
6. Serve and enjoy.

Chicken 'Zoodle' Soup

Serving Yields Provided: 2
Macro Counts - Each Serving:
- Net Carbs: 4 g
- Total Fats: 16 g
- Protein: 34 g
- Calories: 310

Ingredients Needed:
- Chicken broth (3 cups)
- Chicken breast (1)

- Avocado oil (2 tbsp.)
- Green onion (1)
- Celery stalk (1)
- Cilantro (.25 cup)
- Salt (to taste)
- Peeled zucchini (1)

Directions for Preparation:
1. Chop or dice the breast of the chicken. Pour the oil into a saucepan and cook the chicken until done. Pour in the broth and simmer. Chop the celery and green onions and toss into the pan. Simmer for 3 to 4 more minutes.
2. Chop the cilantro and prepare the zucchini noodles. Use a spiralizer or potato peeler to make the 'noodles.' Add to the pot.
3. Simmer for a few more minutes and season to your liking.
4. Store the leftovers in a glass container in the fridge for 2 to 3 days.

Creamy Chicken Soup

Serving Yields Provided: 4
Macro Counts - Each Serving:
- Net Carbs: 2 g
- Total Fats: 25 g
- Protein: 18 g
- Calories: 307

Ingredients Needed:
- Butter (2 tbsp.)
- Large breast of chicken (1–2 cups, shredded)
- Cubed cream cheese (4 oz.)
- Garlic seasoning (2 tbsp.)
- Chicken broth (14.5 oz.)
- Salt (to your liking)
- Heavy cream (.25 cup)

Directions for Preparation:
1. Warm a saucepan and melt the butter using the medium heat setting.

2. Add the shredded chicken and toss. Blend in the cream cheese and seasoning, mixing well.
3. When melted, add the heavy cream and broth.
4. Once boiling, lower the heat and cook slowly for 3 to 4 minutes. Season as desired.

No-Cook Chilled Avocado & Mint Soup

Serving Yields Provided: 2
Macro Counts - Each Serving:
- Net Carbs: 4 g
- Total Fats: 26 g
- Protein: 4 g
- Calories: 280

Ingredients Needed:
- Romaine lettuce (2 leaves)
- Ripened avocado (1 medium)
- Coconut milk (1 cup)
- Lime juice (1 tbsp.)
- Fresh mint (20 leaves)
- Salt (to your liking)

Directions for Preparation:
1. Combine all of the fixings into a blender and mix well. (You want it thick but not like a puree.)
2. Chill in the refrigerator for 5 to 10 minutes before serving.

Seafood

Alfredo Shrimp

Serving Yields Provided: 4
Macro Counts - Each Serving:
- Net Carbs: 6.5 g
- Total Fats: 18 g
- Protein: 23 g
- Calories: 298

Ingredients Needed:
- Raw shrimp (1 lb.)

- Salted butter (1 tbsp.)
- Cubed cream cheese (4 oz.)
- Whole milk (.5 cup)
- Dried basil (1 tsp.)
- Salt (1 tsp.)
- Garlic powder (1 tbsp.)
- Shredded parmesan cheese (.5 cup)
- Baby kale or spinach (.25 cup)
- Whole sun-dried tomatoes (5)
- *Also Needed:* Food processor or blender

Directions for Preparation:

1. Heat the butter using the medium heat setting in a skillet.
2. Toss in the shrimp and lower the heat to medium-low.
3. After 30 seconds, flip the shrimp and cook until slightly pink. Blend in the cream cheese.
4. Increase the heat, and pour in the milk. Stir frequently.
5. Sprinkle with the salt, basil, and garlic. Empty the parmesan cheese in and mix well.
6. Simmer until the sauce has thickened. Cut the sun-dried tomatoes into strips.
7. Lastly, fold in the kale/spinach and sun-dried tomatoes. Serve steaming hot.

Avocado & Salmon Omelet Wrap

Serving Yields Provided: 2
Macro Counts - Each Serving:
- Net Carbs: 5.8 g
- Total Fats: 66.9 g
- Protein: 36.9 g
- Calories: 765

Ingredients Needed:
- Large eggs (3)
- Smoked salmon (1.8 oz.)
- Avocado (.5 of 1 average-size)
- Spring onion (1)

- Cream cheese - full-fat (2 tbsp.)
- Chives, freshly chopped (2 tbsp.)
- Butter or ghee (1 tbsp.)
- Pepper and salt (as desired)

Directions for Preparation:

1. Add a sprinkle of pepper and salt to the eggs. Use a fork or whisk, mixing them well. Blend in the chives and cream cheese.
2. Prepare the salmon and avocado (peel and slice or chop).
3. Combine the butter/ghee and the egg mixture in a frying pan. Continue cooking on low heat until done.
4. Place the omelet on a serving dish with a portion of cheese over it. Sprinkle the onion, prepared avocado, and salmon into the wrap.
5. Close and serve!

Fish Cakes

Serving Yields Provided: 6
Macro Counts - Each Serving:
- Net Carbs: 0.6 g
- Protein: 1.1 g
- Total Fats: 6.5 g
- Calories: 69

Ingredients Needed:
- Wild-caught, raw, and white boneless fish (1 lb.)
- Cilantro, leaves & stems (.25 cup)
- Pinch of salt (1 pinch)
- Chili flakes (1 pinch)
- Coconut oil or grass-fed ghee, for frying (1-2 tbsp.)
- Avocado or neutral oil, for greasing your hands (as needed)
- Avocados (2 ripe)
- Lemon (1 juiced)
- Salt (1 pinch)
- Water (2 tbsp.)
- *Optional*: Garlic cloves (1-2)

- *Also Needed*: Blender or small food processor

Directions for Preparation:
1. In a food processor, add the fish, herbs, garlic (if using), salt, chili, and fish. Blitz until everything is combined evenly.
2. Use the medium-high heat setting on the stovetop to warm a skillet. Add the ghee or coconut oil. Swirl the pan to coat.
3. Put some oil in your hands, and roll the fish mixture into 6 patties.
4. Add the cakes to the heated frying pan. Fry on each side until golden brown.
5. While the fish cakes are cooking, add all of the dipping sauce ingredients (starting with the lemon juice) into the blender. Blitz until smooth and creamy.
6. When the fish cakes are cooked, serve warm with dipping sauce. Taste the fish, and add more lemon juice or salt to your liking.

Lobster Salad

Serving Yields Provided: 4
Macro Counts - Each Serving:
- Net Carbs: 2 g
- Total Fats: 25 g
- Protein: 18 g
- Calories: 307

Ingredients Needed:
- Melted butter (.25 cup)
- Cooked lobster meat (1 lb.)
- Mayonnaise (.25 cup)
- Black pepper (.125 tsp.)

Directions for Preparation:
1. Chop the lobster into bite-sized pieces.

2. Melt and pour the butter over the meat. Toss to coat, and blend in the mayonnaise, along with the pepper.
3. Chill in a covered dish for a minimum of 10 minutes or chill to your liking.

Other Delicious Lunchtime Choices

Buffalo Cauliflower Bites

Serving Yields Provided: 4
Macro Counts - Each Serving:
- Net Carbs: 3 g
- Total Fats: 12 g
- Protein: 2 g
- Calories: 130

Ingredients Needed:
- Cauliflower florets (4 cups)
- Cracked black pepper (as desired)
- Sea salt (.25 tsp.)
- Cayenne pepper (.25 tsp.)
- Salted butter (4 tbsp.)
- Hot sauce (.25 cup)
- Minced garlic (1 clove)
- Paprika (.25 tsp.)
- *Optional:* Blue cheese dressing

Directions for Preparation:
1. Warm the oven until it reaches 375° Fahrenheit.
2. Arrange the florets on a paper-lined baking tray.
3. Whisk the cayenne, black pepper, salt, paprika, garlic, butter, and hot sauce. Pour into a microwavable-safe dish for 30 seconds or until smooth.
4. Empty the sauce over the florets in the pan and bake for 25 minutes.
5. Serve with a bowl of blue cheese dressing for dipping.

Chinese Sauce Fried Rice

Serving Yields Provided:
Macro Counts - Each Serving:
- Net Carbs: 4.3 g Protein: 17 g
- Total Fats: 20.5 g Calories: 289

Ingredients Needed:
- Cauliflower (1 medium head)
- Butter (.5 of 1 stick, 4 tbsp.)
- Green onions (2 large)
- Garlic (4 cloves)
- Carrot (.5 cup)
- Yellow & red bell pepper (.5 cup of each)
- Coconut aminos (4 tbsp.)
- Sesame oil (1 tbsp.)
- Sea salt (1 tsp. or more to your liking)
- Crushed red pepper flakes (.5 tsp.)
- Chinese sausage (.5 lb.)
- Frozen peas (.5 cup)
- Large eggs (3)
- *Also Needed*: Box grater or food processor & Wok

Directions for Preparation:
1. Separately chop the white and green parts of the onions. Mince the garlic cloves and dice the peppers. Thinly slice the carrots and sausage.
2. Rice the cauliflower.
3. Warm up the wok using the medium heat setting. In the wok, warm up 1 tablespoon of butter, garlic, and white portion of the onions. Sauté for 2 to 3 minutes.
4. Toss in the rest of the butter, carrot, and bell peppers. Sauté for 5 to 7 minutes.
5. Toss in the sea salt, red pepper flakes, riced cauliflower, coconut aminos, and sesame oil.
6. Stir-fry for about 10 minutes and add the sausage and peas. Stir-fry for another 5 minutes.
7. Push all the fixings in the wok over to one side.
8. Whisk the eggs using a fork and add to the empty side and lightly scramble. Slowly mix them in with the rest of the fixings.
9. Garnish with green onions and serve.

Mixed Vegetable Patties – Kitchen robot

Serving Yields Provided: 4
Macro Counts - Each Serving:
- Net Carbs: 3 g
- Total Fats: 10 g Protein: 4 g
- Calories: 220

Ingredients Needed:
- Cauliflower florets (1 cup)
- Frozen vegetables (1 bag, mixed)
- Water (1.5 cups)
- Flax meal (1 cup)
- Olive oil (2 tbsp.)

Directions for Preparation:
1. Fill the Kitchen robot with the water, and add the veggies to the steamer basket. Secure the lid and set the timer for 4 to 5 minutes using the high-pressure setting.
2. Quick-release the pressure and drain.
3. Use a potato masher, stirring in the flax meal. Shape into four patties.
4. Select the sauté function in a clean pot and pour in the oil.
5. Prepare the patties until they are golden brown or for about 3 minutes per side before serving.

Pesto Roasted Cabbage & Mushrooms

Serving Yields Provided: 2
Macro Counts - Each Serving:
- Net Carbs: 8 g
- Total Fats: 56 g
- Protein: 13 g
- Calories: 576

Ingredients Needed:
- Shredded cabbage (.75 cup)
- Pesto sauce (2 tbsp.)
- Hard cheese, Italian style, grated (.2 tbsp.)
- Feta cheese (.25 cup crumbled)
- Chopped basil (1 tbsp.)
- Chopped white mushrooms (.25 cup)
- Olive oil (2 tbsp.)

Directions for Preparation:
1. Warm up the oven in advance to 375° Fahrenheit.
2. Prepare the mushrooms and cabbage and arrange on a baking tray.
3. Spritz with oil and toss evenly.
4. Scoop some pesto sauce on top and toss again.
5. Add the grated cheese over the top and bake for about 20 minutes.
6. Serve with a portion of crumbled feta and basil.

Sloppy Joes – Vegan

Serving Yields Provided: 6
Macro Counts - Each Serving:
- Net Carbs: 8.9 g
- Total Fats: 29.9 g
- Protein: 14.7 g
- Calories: 354

Ingredients Needed:
- Hulled hemp seeds (.5 cup)
- Hulled pumpkin seeds - Pepitas (1 cup)
- Chopped walnuts (1 cup)
- Apple cider vinegar (1 tbsp.)
- Prepared mustard (1 tbsp.)
- Tomato paste (6 oz.)
- Garlic powder (.5 tbsp.)
- Onion powder (1 tsp.)
- Granulated sweetener (1 tbsp.)
- Vegetable broth (2 cups)
- Lettuce wraps, for serving

Directions for Preparation:
1. Combine each of the fixings in a dutch oven or soup pot on medium-low heat.
2. Place the top of the pot. Simmer slowly for about 45 minutes, occasionally stirring until the vegetable broth is completely absorbed.
3. Serve on keto rolls or bread.

Chapter 29:

Tasty Dinner Choices

Poultry

Buffalo Chicken Burgers

Serving Yields Provided: 2 burgers
Macro Counts - Each Serving:
- Net Carbs: 1 g
- Total Fats: 34 g
- Protein: 43 g
- Calories: 488

Ingredients Needed:
- Cooked chicken breasts (8 oz.)
- Room-temperature cream cheese (2 oz.)
- Shredded mozzarella cheese (.5 cup)
- Frank's Red-Hot Sauce or your choice (2 tbsp.)
- *For Frying*: Ghee or Coconut oil

Directions for Preparation:
1. Either chop or shred the prepared chicken and combine with the rest of the fixings.
2. Place the fixings in the microwave for 15 to 20 seconds to help compact the ingredients. Form two medium patties and place on a plate. Store in the freezer for about 15 minutes.
3. Warm a skillet using the high heat setting. Add the fat and patties. Cook the burgers for 2 to 3 minutes per side.
4. Serve when crispy brown.

Chicken & Asparagus

Serving Yields Provided: 8
Macro Counts - Each Serving:
- Net Carbs: 4 g Total Fats: 18.2 g
- Protein: 63 g Calories: 439

Ingredients Needed:
- Chicken breasts (4 lb.)
- Avocado oil (1 tbsp.)
- Trimmed asparagus (1 lb.)
- Sun-dried tomatoes (4)
- Thick-cut bacon (4 slices)
- Salt (1 tsp.)
- Pepper (.25 tsp.)
- Provolone cheese (8 slices)
- *Also Needed*: 1 baking pan

Directions for Preparation:
1. Set the oven temperature to 400° Fahrenheit.
2. Cut the chicken breasts into eight thin pieces. Chop the bacon and tomatoes into one-inch pieces.
3. Add the oil to the baking pan, along with the chicken and asparagus. Top it off with the tomatoes and bacon.
4. Sprinkle some pepper and salt for seasoning.
5. Bake until the chicken reaches 160° Fahrenheit (internally) or about 25 minutes.
6. Toss in the asparagus and cheese.
7. Garnish with a portion of bacon and tomatoes.
8. Bake for another 3 to 4 minutes until the cheese has melted.

Chicken BBQ Zucchini Boats

Serving Yields Provided: 4
Macro Counts - Each Serving:
- Net Carbs: 9 g
- Total Fats: 11 g
- Protein: 19 g
- Calories: 212

Ingredients Needed:
- Zucchini (3 halved)
- Boneless skinless chicken breast (1 lb. cooked and shredded)
- BBQ sauce (.5 cup)
- Shredded Mexican cheese (.33 cup)
- Avocado (1 sliced)
- Halved cherry tomatoes (.5 cup)
- Diced green onions (.25 cup)
- Keto-friendly ranch dressing (3 tbsp. to drizzle)
- *Also Needed:* 9x13 casserole dish

Directions for Preparation:
1. Warm up the oven to 350° Fahrenheit.
2. Scoop the seeds out of the zucchini halves, leaving a ½-inch hole carved out of the center (similar to a boat). Place the zucchini flesh side up into the casserole dish.
3. Add shredded chicken and BBQ sauce to a small bowl. Toss to coat all the chicken with the barbeque sauce.
4. Fill the zucchini boats with the BBQ chicken mixture. (about .25 to .33 cup for each zucchini boat)
5. Sprinkle with Mexican cheese on top.
6. Bake for 15 minutes. (Note: If you would like it to be more tender, bake for an additional 5 to 10 minutes to your desired tenderness)
7. Remove from oven.
8. Garnish with avocado, tomatoes, green onion, and a drizzle of ranch dressing. Serve.

Roasted Chicken & Tomatoes

Serving Yields Provided: 2
Macro Counts - Each Serving:
- Net Carbs: 5 g
- Protein: 16 g
- Total Fats: 16 g
- Calories: 233

Ingredients Needed:
- Olive oil (1 tbsp.)
- Plum tomatoes (2 quartered)
- Chicken legs, bone-in with skin (2)
- Paprika (1 tsp.)
- Ground oregano (1 tsp.)
- Balsamic vinegar (1 tbsp.)

Directions for Preparation:
1. Set the oven temperature setting to 350° Fahrenheit. Grease a roasting pan with a spritz of oil.
2. Rinse and lightly dab the chicken legs dry with a paper towel. Prepare using the oil and vinegar over the skin. Season with paprika and oregano.
3. Arrange the legs in the pan, along with the tomatoes around the edges.
4. Cover with a layer of foil and bake for 1 hour. Baste to prevent the chicken from drying out.
5. Discard the foil and increase the temperature to 425° Fahrenheit.
6. Bake 15 to 30 minutes more until browned and the juices run clear.
7. Serve with a side salad.

Sesame Chicken Egg Roll in a Bowl

Serving Yields Provided: 8
Macro Counts - Each Serving:
- Net Carbs: 3.3 g
- Protein: 15 g
- Total Fats: 19.5 g
- Calories: 267

Ingredients Needed:

- Toasted sesame oil (3 tbsp.)
- Red onion (1 small, about .5 cup)
- Garlic (4 cloves)minced
- Green onions (5)
- Boneless chicken breast or thigh (1.5 lb.)
- Black pepper (.5 tsp.)
- Sea salt (1 tsp.)
- Ginger powder (1 tsp.)
- Sriracha sauce or garlic chili sauce (1 tbsp. + 1 tsp.)
- Broccoli slaw (20 oz.)
- Unseasoned rice vinegar (2 tbsp.)
- Coconut aminos (.25 cup)
- Toasted sesame seeds (1 tbsp.)

Directions for Preparation:

1. Chop the red onion and slice the onions on the bias (separate the white and green portions). Mince the garlic. Cut the chicken into bite-sized pieces.
2. Warm up the oil in a large pan using the medium-high temperature setting.
3. Toss in the garlic, red onion, and white portion of the green onions into the skillet. Sauté until the onions are translucent and the garlic is fragrant.
4. Add the chicken, salt, pepper, ginger, and Sriracha to the pan. Sauté until it's fully cooked.
5. Add the aminos, broccoli slaw, and vinegar. Sauté until the broccoli is tender.
6. Garnish the dish using the green parts of the onions, and sesame seeds before serving. Add Sriracha sauce as desired.

Pork

BBQ Pork Loin

Serving Yields Provided: 4
Macro Counts - Each Serving:

- Net Carbs: 3 g
- Total Fats: 8 g
- Protein: 35 g
- Calories: 238

Ingredients Needed:

- Pork loin (1 lb.)
- Tomato paste (4 tbsp.)
- Worcestershire sauce (1 tsp.)
- Avocado oil (2 tbsp.)
- Smoked paprika (.5 tsp.)
- Minced garlic (.5 tsp.)
- Chopped onion (1 tbsp.)

Directions for Preparation:

1. Whisk the minced garlic, chopped onion, paprika, tomato paste, and Worcestershire sauce.
2. Use the rub to prepare the pork and wrap in foil.
3. Marinate the pork loin in the fridge for at least 1/2 hour for the spices to be absorbed.
4. Add the trivet to the Kitchen robot, and pour the water into the cooker. Secure the lid.
5. Set the timer to 60 minutes. Release the pressure naturally when it's done.
6. Serve.

Carnitas – Crockpot

Serving Yields Provided: 2
Macro Counts - Each Serving:

- Net Carbs: 4 g
- Total Fats: 26 g
- Protein: 45 g
- Calories: 446

Ingredients Needed:
- Boneless pork butt roast (1 lb.)
- Chili powder (.5 tbsp.)
- Olive oil (1 tbsp.)
- Small diced onion (.5 of 1)
- Minced cloves of garlic (2)
- Juiced lime (1 whole lime)
- Black pepper and Pink salt (as desired)

Directions for Preparation:
1. Use the low-temperature setting to warm up the crockpot.
2. Whisk the olive oil with the chili powder. Rub over the pork and place in the cooker, the fatty side facing up.
3. Prepare the veggies and add along with the lime juice, salt, and pepper.
4. Place the lid on the pot and simmer on low for 8 hours.
5. When ready, shred the meat on a cutting board using two forks.
6. Enjoy on a leaf of lettuce, but remember to add any additional carbs to the carb count.
7. Total prep is just 10 minutes with a cooking time of 8 hrs.

Crack Slaw – Pork Egg Roll in a Bowl

Serving Yields Provided: 4
Macro Counts - Each Serving:
- Net Carbs: 5.5 g
- Protein: 20 g
- Total Fats: 20 g
- Calories: 297

Ingredients Needed:
- Sesame oil (2 tbsp.)
- Garlic (3 cloves)
- Yellow onion (.5 cup)
- Green onions, white and green parts (5)
- Ground pork (1 lb.)
- Ground ginger (.5 tsp.)

- Sea salt & black pepper (as desired)
- Sriracha or garlic chili sauce (1 tbsp.)
- Rice vinegar (1 tbsp.)
- Coleslaw mix (14 oz. bag)
- Coconut Aminos (3 tbsp.)
- Toasted sesame seeds (2 tbsp.)

Directions for Preparation:
1. Mince the garlic, and dice the yellow onion. Slice the green onions on the bias.
2. Warm up the oil in a skillet using the medium-high temperature setting.
3. Toss the garlic, white portion of the green onions, and the yellow onions into the pan. Sauté until the onions are translucent and the garlic is fragrant.
4. Add the ground pork, sea salt, black pepper, ground ginger, and Sriracha. Sauté until the pork is fully cooked.
5. Add the coconut aminos, coleslaw mix, and vinegar. Sauté until the coleslaw is tender.
6. Garnish with green onions and sesame seeds before serving.

Pan-Fried Chops

Serving Yields Provided: 3
Macro Counts - Each Serving:
- Net Carbs: 4.2 g
- Total Fats: 27 g
- Protein: 22 g
- Calories: 385

Ingredients Needed:
- Coconut flour (.5 cup)
- Salt and black pepper (1 tsp. each)
- Pork chops (3)
- Butter (1 tbsp.)

Directions for Preparation:
1. Combine all of the dry fixings in a large mixing container.
2. Pat the chops dry with a paper towel.
3. Melt the butter in a skillet on the stovetop.

4. Cover the chops with the mixture and prepare each side for 4 to 5 minutes.
5. Serve with your favorite side dishes.

Parmesan Crusted Pork Chops

Serving Yields Provided: 14
Macro Counts - Each Serving:
- Net Carbs: 3 g
- Total Fats: 34 g
- Protein: 33 g
- Calories: 354

Ingredients Needed:
- Parmesan cheese (6 oz.)
- Pork chops (14)
- Large eggs (2)
- Almond flour (.75 cup)
- Pepper and salt (to taste)
- *For Frying:* Bacon grease

Directions for Preparation:
1. Heat the oven to 400° Fahrenheit.
2. Grate the parmesan and mix with the flour and spices.
3. Whisk the eggs in a shallow dish.
4. Dip the chops in the eggs and then the parmesan mixture.
5. Fry on each side using the bacon grease for 1 minute.
6. Arrange on a baking dish in the oven, baking until done. Serve.

Slow-Cooked Kalua Pork & Cabbage

Serving Yields Provided: 12
Macro Counts - Each Serving:
- Net Carbs: 4 g
- Total Fats: 13 g
- Protein: 22 g
- Calories: 227

Ingredients Needed:
- Boneless pork shoulder butt (3 lb.)
- Head of cabbage (1 medium, approx. 2 lb.)
- Bacon (7 strips, divided)
- Coarse sea salt (1 tbsp.)
- *Suggested*: 6-quart slow cooker

Directions for Preparation:
1. Coarsely chop the cabbage. Trim the fat from the roast.
2. Layer most of the bacon in the cooker. Dust the salt over the roast and place the rest of the bacon on top. Close the top and cook on low for 8 to 10 hours.
3. At that time, drop in the cabbage and continue cooking, covered for another hour until it's tender (time may vary).
4. When the roast is done, remove, and shred. Use a slotted spoon to arrange the cabbage in the serving dish.
5. Use some of the slow cooker juices on the side for dipping.

Stuffed Pork Tenderloin on the Grill

Serving Yields Provided: 6
Macro Counts - Each Serving:
- Net Carbs: 3 g
- Total Fats: 6 g
- Protein: 29 g
- Calories: 194

Ingredients Needed:
- Pork tenderloin or venison (2 lb.)
- Feta cheese (.5 cup)
- Gorgonzola cheese (.5 cup)
- Onion (1 tsp.)
- Cloves of garlic (2 cloves)
- Crushed almonds (2 tbsp.)
- Sea Salt & black pepper (.5 tsp. each)

Directions for Preparation:
1. Warm up the grill.

2. Create a pocket in the tenderloin using a sharp knife.
3. Chop the onion and mince the garlic.
4. Combine the cheeses, onions, almonds, and garlic.
5. Stuff the pork pocket and seal using a skewer.
6. Grill until done (approx. 1 hr.) with the lid closed (about 300-350° Fahrenheit).
7. The center of the meat should reach 150° Fahrenheit.
8. Cover it with foil, and let it rest for about 15 minutes before serving.

Fish Seafood Options

Baked Tilapia With Cherry Tomatoes

Serving Yields Provided: 2
Macro Counts - Each Serving:
- Net Carbs: 4 g
- Total Fats: 8 g
- Protein: 23 g
- Calories: 180

Ingredients Needed:
- Lemon juice (1 tbsp.)
- Butter (2 tsp.)
- Tilapia fillets (2, 4 oz. each)
- Cherry tomatoes (8)
- Pitted black olives (.25 cup)
- Black pepper (.25 tsp.)
- Paprika (.25 tsp.)
- Garlic powder (1 tsp.)
- Salt (.5 tsp.)
- *Optional*: Balsamic vinegar (1 tbsp.)

Directions for Preparation:
1. Set the oven to 375° Fahrenheit.
2. Lightly spritz a roasting pan with some cooking oil. Add the butter, along with the olives and tomatoes in the bottom.

3. Season the tilapia with the spices (paprika, salt, pepper, and garlic powder).
4. Lastly, add the fish fillets with the freshly squeezed lemon juice.
5. Cover the pan with foil and bake until the fish easily flakes (25 to 30 minutes).
6. Garnish with the vinegar if desired.

Chili Lime Cod

Serving Yields Provided: 2
Macro Counts - Each Serving:
- Net Carbs: 3 g
- Total Fats: 5 g
- Protein: 37 g
- Calories: 215

Ingredients Needed:
- Wild-caught cod (10–12 oz.)
- Coconut flour (.33 cup)
- Egg (3)
- Lime (1)
- Garlic powder (1 tsp.)
- Cayenne pepper (.5 tsp.)
- Salt (1 tsp.)
- Crushed red pepper (1 tsp.)

Directions for Preparation:
1. Heat the oven temperature to reach 400° Fahrenheit.
2. In separate dishes, whip the egg and remove any lumps from the flour.
3. Let the fillet soak in the egg dish for 1 minute on each side. Add it to the flour dish, and then add it to a baking sheet.
4. Sprinkle the spices and drizzle the lime juice over the cod.
5. Bake it for 10 to 12 minutes or when it easily flakes apart.
6. Drizzle with some Sriracha if you wish, and enjoy.

Lemon Shrimp

Serving Yields Provided: 2
Macro Counts - Each Serving:
- Net Carbs: 2.5 g
- Total Fats: 27 g
- Protein: 22.5 g
- Calories: 335

Ingredients Needed:
- Olive oil (.25 cup)
- Large shrimp (.5 lb.)
- Garlic cloves (3)
- Lemon (1 wedge)
- Pepper and salt (as desired)

Directions for Preparation:
1. Sauté the garlic with the cayenne along with the olive oil using medium heat.
2. Peel the shrimp and cook 2–3 minutes per side.
3. Dust the shrimp with the pepper, salt, and a lemon wedge.
4. Use the remainder of the garlic oil for a dipping sauce.

Skillet Fried Cod

Serving Yields Provided:
Macro Counts - Each Serving: 4
- Net Carbs: 1 g
- Total Fats: 7 g
- Protein: 21 g
- Calories: 160

Ingredients Needed:
- Ghee (3 tbsp.)
- Cod fillets (4, .33 lb. ea.)
- Minced garlic cloves (6)
- *Optional:* Garlic powder
- *Optional:* Salt

Directions for Preparation:
1. Melt the ghee, and add half of the garlic into a skillet.

2. Arrange the fillets in the pan using medium-high heat. Sprinkle with garlic, pepper, and salt.
3. Once it turns white halfway up its side, turn it over, and add the remainder of the minced garlic. Continue cooking until it flakes easily.
4. Serve with some ghee/garlic from the pan.

Beef Options

Bacon Cheeseburger

Serving Yields Provided: 12
Macro Counts - Each Serving:
- Net Carbs: 0.8 g
- Protein: 27 g
- Total Fats: 41 g
- Calories: 489

Ingredients Needed:
- Low-sodium bacon (16 oz. pkg.)
- Ground beef (3 lb.)
- Eggs (2)
- Medium chopped onion (.5 of 1)
- Shredded cheddar cheese (8 oz.)

Directions for Preparation:
1. Fry the bacon, and chop it into bits. Shred the cheese, and dice the onion.
2. Combine the mixture with the beef and blend in the whisked eggs.
3. Prepare 24 burgers, and grill them the way you like them.
4. You can make a double-decker since they are small. If you like a larger burger, you can just make 12 burgers as a single-decker.

Barbacoa Beef – Kitchen robot

Serving Yields Provided: 9
Macro Counts - Each Serving:
- Net Carbs: 2 g
- Total Fats: 4.5 g
- Protein: 24 g
- Calories: 153

Ingredients Needed:
- Eye round/bottom round roast (3 lb.)
- Black pepper (as desired)
- Kosher salt (2.5 tsp.)
- Water (1 cup)
- Medium onion (0.5 of 1)
- Lime (1 juiced)
- Garlic cloves (5)
- Chipotles in adobo sauce (2–4)
- Oregano (1 tbsp.)
- Ground cumin (1 tbsp.)
- Oil (1 tsp.)
- Bay leaves (3)
- Ground cloves (0.5 tsp.)

Directions for Preparation:
1. Program the Kitchen robot using the sauté function.
2. Cut the fat from the beef and slice into three-inch segments. Sprinkle with pepper and salt.
3. In a blender, puree the water, cloves, chipotles, oregano, lime juice, onion, garlic, and cumin. Pour in the oil, and brown the meat for about 5 minutes. Add the sauce (from the blender) and the bay leaves.
4. Cook for 65 minutes (sauté mode with the top on) until it's easily shredded with two forks. Add water if needed to ensure it remains moist.
5. When ready, arrange on a serving platter, shred, and add it back to the pot. Save the juices for later and remove the bay leaves.
6. Measure 1.5 cups of the reserved juices, and put 1/2 of a teaspoon of cumin and salt.
7. Serve once it has warmed up and the flavors have blended.

BBQ Flank Steak

Serving Yields Provided: 8
Macro Counts - Each Serving:
- Net Carbs: 1 g
- Total Fats: 21 g
- Protein: 35 g
- Calories: 342

Ingredients Needed:
- Flank steak (3 lb.)
- Paprika (1 tsp.)
- Granulated garlic (1 tsp.)
- Cayenne pepper (1 tsp.)
- Granulated onion (1 tsp.)
- White pepper (1 tsp.)
- Salt (1 tsp.)
- Black pepper (1 tsp.)
- Coconut aminos (1 tbsp.)
- Water (.25 cup)
- Melted butter (2 tbsp.)

Directions for Preparation:
1. Combine the aminos, seasonings, and melted butter. Rub into the steak.
2. Add the water to the cooker and the steak fixings.
3. Cook it for 8 hours, flipping halfway through the cooking cycle.
4. Serve with some creamy spinach.

Cheeseburger Calzones

Serving Yields Provided: 8
Macro Counts - Each Serving:
- Net Carbs: 3 g
- Total Fats: 47 g
- Protein: 34 g
- Calories: 580

Ingredients Needed:

- Dill pickle spears (4)
- Cream cheese - divided (8 oz.)
- Shredded mozzarella cheese (1 cup)
- Egg (1) - Almond flour (1 cup)
- Lean ground beef (1.5 lb.)
- Yellow diced onion (.5 of 1)
- Thick-cut bacon strips (4)
- Mayonnaise (.5 cup)
- Shredded cheddar cheese (1 cup)

Directions for Preparation:

1. Program the oven to 425° Fahrenheit.
2. Prepare a cookie tin with parchment paper.
3. Chop the pickles into spears. Set aside for now.
4. Prepare the crust. Combine half of the cream cheese and mozzarella cheese. Microwave for 35 seconds. When it melts, add the egg and almond flour to make the dough. Set aside.
5. Cook the beef on the stove using medium heat. Cook the bacon using the microwave or stovetop for 5 minutes. When it has cooled, break it into bits.
6. Dice the onion and add to the beef. Cook it until softened. Toss in the bacon, cheddar cheese, pickle bits, the rest of the cream cheese, and mayonnaise. Stir well.
7. Roll the dough onto the prepared baking tin. Scoop the mixture into the center. Fold the ends and sides to make the calzone.
8. Bake it until browned or for about 15 minutes. Let it rest for 10 minutes before slicing.

Enchilada

Serving Yields Provided: 4
Macro Counts - Each Serving:
- Net Carbs: 7 g Total Fats: 30 g
- Protein: 36 g Calories: 455

Ingredients Needed:

- Small yellow onion (1)
- Ground beef (1.5 lb.)
- Red enchilada sauce (.66 cup)
- Chopped green onions (8)
- Diced Roma tomatoes (2)
- Shredded cheddar cheese (4 oz.)
- *Optional*: Freshly chopped cilantro (as desired)

Directions for Preparation:

1. Use a wok or skillet to sauté the yellow onion and meat.
2. Drain the juices and fold in the green onions, tomato, and enchilada sauce.
3. Once it starts to boil, simmer for about 5 minutes. Sprinkle with salt and cheese. Continue cooking until the cheese has melted.
4. Stir in the cilantro. Serve over chopped lettuce and a serving of sour cream. Add the extra carbs and enjoy.

Ground Beef Vegetable Skillet

Serving Yields Provided:
Macro Counts - Each Serving:
- Net Carbs: g
- Total Fats: g
- Protein: g
- Calories:

Ingredients Needed:

- Extra virgin olive oil (2 tbsp.)
- Grass-fed, extra-lean ground beef (1 lb.)
- Clove of garlic (1)
- Onions (.5 cup)
- Red bell peppers (.5 cup)
- Zucchini (1 medium)
- Asparagus (.5 lb.)
- Dijon mustard (1 tsp.)
- Tomato passata or tomato sauce (.25 cup)
- Dried oregano (.5 tsp.)

- *Optional*: Crushed red pepper (.125 tsp.)
- Salt and freshly ground black pepper (as desired)
- *For the Garnish*:
- Freshly chopped parsley (to your liking)
- Crumbled feta cheese (1 tbsp.)

Directions for Preparation:

1. Mince or dice the garlic, onions, and peppers. Quarter the zucchini, and slice the asparagus into three segments each.
2. Warm up a large skillet using the medium-high heat setting, and add the olive oil
3. Toss in the garlic and beef. Break apart as it cooks. Stir it occasionally and cook for about 7 minutes until it's no longer pink. Remove the meat from the skillet, and set it aside for now.
4. Fold in the onions and red bell peppers. Simmer until the onions are softened or about 3 to 4 minutes. Pour in a little bit of olive oil to help sauté the veggies as needed.
5. Toss in the zucchini and asparagus. Simmer for another 3 to 5 minutes.
6. Return the beef to the skillet, and mix everything together.
7. Simmer for one to two additional minutes.

Hamburger Stroganoff

Serving Yields Provided: 1
Macro Counts - Each Serving:
- Net Carbs: 6 g
- Total Fats: 28 g
- Protein: 39 g
- Calories: 447

Ingredients Needed:
- Lean ground beef (1 lb.)

- Sliced mushrooms (8 oz.)
- Minced cloves of garlic (2)
- Butter (2 tbsp.)
- Sour cream (1.25 cups)
- Water or dry white wine (.33 cup)
- Lemon juice (1 tsp.)
- Dried parsley (1 tsp.)
- Paprika (.25 tsp.)
- *Optional*: Freshly chopped parsley (1 tbsp.)

Directions for Preparation:

1. Warm a skillet to sauté the onions and garlic using 1 tbsp butter.
2. Mix the beef into the pan and sprinkle with pepper and salt if desired. Cook until done and set to the side.
3. Add the remainder of the butter, mushrooms, and the wine or water to the pan. Cook until half of the liquid is reduced and the mushrooms are soft.
4. Take it away from the heat, and add the paprika and sour cream.
5. On low heat, stir in the meat and lemon juice. Use additional spices for flavoring if desired.

Mongolian Beef

Serving Yields Provided: 6
Macro Counts - Each Serving:
- Net Carbs: 1.99 g
- Total Fats: 19 g
- Protein: 37 g
- Calories: 339

Ingredients Needed:
- Flank steak (1.5 lb.)
- *Optional:* Crushed red pepper flakes (.25 tsp.)
- Fish sauce (1 tbsp.)
- Garlic cloves (3)
- Toasted sesame oil (2 tbsp.)
- Gluten-free coconut aminos (2 tbsp.)
- Golden monk fruit sweetener, e.g., Lakanto (.5 cup)

- Avocado oil (1 tbsp.)
- Fresh ginger (1 tbsp.)
- Glucomannan powder or xanthan gum (1.5 tsp.) - Green onions (2 tbsp.)

Directions for Preparation:

1. Mince the cloves of garlic, and grate the piece of ginger. Thinly slice the onions.
2. Cutting against the grain, slice the steak into thin strips then into one to two-inch pieces. Set aside.
3. Whisk the fish sauce, red pepper flakes, minced garlic, aminos, sesame oil, and monk fruit sweetener.
4. Add the sliced steak and rotate steak strips until all meat is coated in marinade. Cover the bowl and transfer to the fridge to marinate for 30 minutes.
5. Once the steak has finished marinating, heat the avocado oil in a skillet using the medium temperature setting. Add the steak, marinade, and grated ginger to the pan. Cook the steak until browned, flipping as needed. Remove from the burner. Spoon out .5 cup of the sauce from the pan and transfer to a mixing bowl. Sprinkle the glucomannan powder on top of the sauce. Whisk the fixings together until the sauce thickens.
6. Pour the sauce back into the pan.
7. Serve the beef in bowls on its own or atop cauliflower rice, and garnish it with sliced green onions.
8. Consume within 2 to 3 days, or freeze it for 2 months.

Nacho Skillet Steak

Serving Yields Provided: 5
Macro Counts - Each Serving:
- Net Carbs: 6 g Total Fats: 31 g
- Protein: 19 g Calories: 385

Ingredients Needed:
- Butter (1 tbsp.)
- Beef round tip steak (8 oz.)
- Melted refined coconut oil (.33 cup)
- Turmeric (.5 tsp.)
- Chili powder (1 tsp.)
- Cauliflower (1.5 lb.)
- Shredded cheddar cheese (1 oz.)
- Shredded Monterey Jack cheese (1 oz.)

Optional Toppings:
- Canned jalapeno slices (1 oz.)
- Sour cream (.33 cup)
- Avocado (5 oz.)

Directions for Preparation:
1. Set the oven temperature to 400° Fahrenheit.
2. Cut the cauliflower into chip-like shapes.
3. Combine the turmeric, chili powder, and coconut oil in a mixing dish.
4. Toss in the cauliflower, and add it to a baking tin. Set the baking timer for 20 to 25 minutes.
5. Over medium-high heat in a cast iron skillet, add the butter. Cook until both sides of the meat is done, flipping just once. Let it rest for 5–10 minutes. Thinly slice and sprinkle with some pepper and salt.
6. When done, transfer the florets to the skillet, and add the steak strips. Top it with the cheese and bake for 5–10 more minutes.
7. Serve with your favorite garnish, but you have to count those carbs.

Slow-Cooked London Broil

Serving Yields Provided: 4
Macro Counts - Each Serving:
- Net Carbs: 2.5 g
- Protein: 47 g
- Total Fats: 18 g
- Calories: 409

Ingredients Needed:
- Minced garlic (2 tsp.)
- London broil (2 lb.)
- Dijon mustard (1 tbsp.)
- Reduced sugar ketchup (2 tbsp.)
- Coconut Aminos/ your choice soy sauce substitute (2 tbsp.)
- Coffee (.5 cup)
- Chicken broth (.5 cup)
- White wine (.25 cup)
- Onion powder (2 tsp.)

Directions for Preparation:

1. Arrange the beef in the cooker. Cover both sides with the mustard, soy sauce, ketchup, and minced garlic.
2. Pour the liquid components into the cooker, and give it a sprinkle of the onion powder.
3. Cook it for 4 to 6 hours.
4. When the timer buzzes, shred the meat. Combine with the juices and serve.

Chapter 30:

Snacktime Treats

Arancini – 5-Cheese Bacon & Cauliflower Bites

Serving Yields Provided: 10, 3 balls each
Macro Counts - Each Serving:
- Net Carbs: 5.4 g Total Fats: 19 g
- Protein: 19 g Calories: 280

Ingredients Needed:
- Riced cauliflower (5 cups)
- Bacon (1 lb.)
- Cream cheese (8 oz.)
- Goat cheese (4 oz.)
- Sharp cheddar cheese (.5 cup)
- Grated parmesan cheese (1.5 cups, divided)
- Sharp garlic & white cheddar cheese (.5 cup)
- Garlic (3 cloves)
- Italian seasoning, divided (1 tsp.)
- Black pepper (.5 tsp.)
- Onion powder (1 tsp.)
- Garlic powder (1 tsp.)
- Crushed pork rinds (1 cup)
- Panko or extra crushed pork rinds (.5 cup)
- Sea salt (.5 tsp.)
- Oil (as needed)

Directions for Preparation:
1. Cook and crumble the bacon. Let the cream cheese sit out a few minutes to soften. Prepare the cauliflower. Pulse it in a food processor or cheese grater. Mince the garlic and crush the pork rinds.
2. Combine the bacon, riced cauliflower, goat cheese, softened cream cheese, sharp cheddar cheese, .5 tsp Italian seasoning, sharp garlic, and white cheddar cheese, .5 cup grated Parmesan, minced garlic, sea salt, and pepper.
3. Combine all of the fixings until incorporated well. Refrigerate for 1 to 2 hours until it's firm.
4. Mix the crushed pork rinds, the rest of the parmesan cheese, panko, the rest of the Italian seasoning, onion powder, and garlic powder for the breading.
5. After the cauliflower mixture has chilled and is firm, roll the mixture into balls. Freeze for 3 hours or overnight.
6. Pour oil, measuring 1-inch thick, and heat it using the medium-high temperature setting.
7. Roll each of the balls in the breading mixture until all balls are evenly coated.
8. When the oil is hot, drop the balls into the pan, and fry the balls, five or six at a time. Fry them until they are evenly browned to your liking.
9. Transfer to a paper-lined platter. Serve.

BBQ Chicken Pizza

Serving Yields Provided: 4
Macro Counts - Each Serving:
- Net Carbs: 6.5 g
- Total Fats: 16 g
- Protein: 24 g
- Calories: 282

Ingredients Needed:
- Parmesan cheese (3 oz.)
- Psyllium husk powder (3 tbsp.)
- Pepper & salt (1-2 pinches)
- Large eggs (6)
- Italian seasoning (1.5 tsp.)
- Shredded chicken (6 oz.)
- Barbecue sauce (4 tbsp.)
- Cheddar cheese (4 oz.)
- Tomato sauce (4 tbsp.)
- Mayonnaise (1 tbsp.)

Directions for Preparation:
1. Heat the oven until it reaches 425° Fahrenheit.
2. Shred the cheese. Combine the psyllium powder, parmesan, eggs, pepper, salt, and Italian seasoning. Once the dough has thickened, arrange it on a parchment paper to fit on a baking tin.
3. Bake it on the top rack of the oven for 10 minutes. Flip the crust, and add the rest of the fixings. Broil on high for 3 minutes and serve.
4. The total time to cook the pizza from start to finish is just 20 minutes.

Chicken Nuggets

Serving Yields Provided: 6
Macro Counts - Each Serving:
- Net Carbs: 2 g
- Total Fats: 17 g
- Protein: 18 g
- Calories: 243

Ingredients Needed:
- Cooked chicken (2 cups)
- Cream cheese (8 oz.)
- Egg (1)
- Garlic salt (1 tsp.)
- Almond flour (.25 cup)

Directions for Preparation:
1. Set the oven temperature to 350° Fahrenheit.
2. Lightly grease a baking pan with a spritz of cooking oil spray. You can also use a layer of parchment paper.
3. Shred the chicken using a food processor or by hand. (Try using a combination of dark and light meat.)
4. Combine the rest of the fixings and mix well.
5. Scoop the nugget mixture onto the baking tin.
6. Bake it until firm and slightly browned (12 to 14 min.).

Chicken Salad Deviled Eggs

Serving Yields Provided: 6
Macro Counts - Each Serving:
- Net Carbs: 2 g
- Total Fats: 7 g
- Protein: 13 g
- Calories: 128

Ingredients Needed:
- Old Bay Seasoning (1 dash)
- Lemon pepper (.5 tsp.)
- Dill (.5 tsp.)
- Celery salt (1 pinch)
- Chopped onion (1 tbsp.)
- Dijon mustard (1 tsp.)
- Mayonnaise (2 tbsp.)
- Shredded chicken (1 cup)
- Eggs (6 large)

Directions for Preparation:
1. Combine all of the fixings, and omit the eggs. Store it in the fridge for later.
2. Gently place the eggs in a pot of water (just enough to cover the eggs).
3. Set the temperature on high until it boils, and then lower the setting to medium.

4. Boil for 15 minutes and transfer to cool under cold running water.
5. Remove the shell, and slice the eggs into halves. Remove the yolk and fill with the salad mixture. Sprinkle with the old bay seasoning.
6. *Note*: Discard the yolks or use in another recipe. Total time is just 30 minutes.

Delicious Grilled Cheese Sandwiches

Serving Yields Provided: 2
Macro Counts - Each Serving:
- Net Carbs: 5 g
- Total Fats: 46 g
- Protein: 116 g
- Calories: 520

Ingredients Needed:
- Unsalted butter, divided (5 tbsp.)
- Whole milk, divided (4 tbsp.)
- Eggs, divided (2 large)
- Salt, divided (.25 tsp.)
- Coconut flour, divided (4 tbsp.)
- Baking powder, divided (1 tsp.)
- Sharp cheddar (2 oz.)

Directions for Preparation:
1. Add 2 tablespoons of butter into the dish. Microwave for about 50 seconds or until melted.
2. Mix in 2 tbsp of milk, 1 egg, and 1/8 tsp salt.
3. Add 2 tbsp coconut flour and 1/2 tsp baking powder. Mix until thoroughly combined.
4. Microwave the butter for 90 seconds. Allow it to rest for a minute.
5. Loosen the edges of the bread from the container. Arrange the bread on a rack to cool. Repeat the steps to make a second slice of keto bread.

6. Warm 1 tablespoon of butter in a skillet using the medium-low temperature setting.
7. Assemble the sandwich by placing two cheese slices between the keto bread slices you just made.
8. Once the butter foams, place the sandwich in the skillet.
9. Bake until the cheese has melted or 3 to 5 minutes on each side using medium-low heat.
10. Press on the sandwich with a large spatula.
11. Put the keto grilled cheese sandwich on a platter, and slice it into two triangles and serve.

Grilled Zucchini & Cheese Sandwich

Serving Yields Provided: 2
Macro Counts - Each Serving:
- Net Carbs: 6 g
- Total Fats: 90.1 g
- Protein: 29 g
- Calories: 936

Ingredients Needed:
- Shredded zucchini (2 cups)
- Egg (1)
- Shredded Italian-style hard cheese (.125 cup)
- Shredded cheddar cheese (.5 cup)
- Green sliced onions, sliced (.25 cup)
- Cornstarch (.25 tbsp.)
- Coconut oil (4 tbsp.)

Directions for Preparation:
1. Shred the zucchini and wrap in towels for about 1 hour. Use a skillet or other heavy object over it to squeeze out the extra liquids.
2. Combine with the egg, cornstarch, cheese, and onions. Sprinkle with pepper and salt. Toss well.
3. Pour oil in a skillet to cover the pan, and warm it using the medium heat

temperature setting. When it's hot, add about ¼ of the zucchini mixture into the skillet, shaping it into a square.

4. Cook it until golden, and drain the grease using paper towels.
5. In the same pan, add two zucchini patties and top with cheddar cheese. Add the second patty on top to make a sandwich.

Pepper Jack Mug Melt

Serving Yields Provided: 1
Macro Counts - Each Serving:
- Net Carbs: 3.83 g
- Total Fats: 18 g
- Protein: 22.4g
- Calories: 268

Ingredients Needed:
- Roast beef deli slices (2 oz.)
- Diced green chiles (1.5 tbsp.)
- Sour cream (1 tbsp.)
- Shredded pepper jack cheese (1.5 oz.)

Directions for Preparation:
1. Tear apart the roast beef, and layer it in the bottom of the dish.
2. First, spread half of the sour cream, followed by a ½ tablespoon of the green chili.
3. Layer it with ½ ounce of the pepper cheese. Follow with another layer.
4. Microwave for 1 to 2 minutes until the cheese melts. Serve.

Smoked Salmon & Cream Cheese Roll-Ups

Serving Yields Provided: 2
Macro Counts - Each Serving:
- Net Carbs: 3 g
- Total Fats: 22 g
- Protein: 14g
- Calories: 268

Ingredients Needed:
- Chopped scallions, green and white parts (2 tbsp.)
- Dijon mustard (1 tsp.)
- Grated lemon zest (1 tsp.)
- Room temperature cream cheese (4 oz.)
- Cold smoked salmon (12 slices, 4 oz.)
- Salt & Freshly ground black pepper (as desired)

Directions for Preparation:
1. In a blender or food processor, add the lemon zest, cream cheese, scallions, and mustard. Flavor with pepper and salt according to taste. Mix until creamy smooth.
2. Spread the cheese mix on both sides of the salmon and roll. Arrange with the seam side down on a platter.
3. Cover it with plastic and place in the fridge until it's ready to eat. They will remain fresh for about 3 days.

Spicy Beef Wraps

Serving Yields Provided: 2
Macro Counts - Each Serving:
- Net Carbs: 4 g
- Total Fats: g
- Protein: 30 g
- Calories: 375

Ingredients Needed:
- Coconut oil (1–2 tbsp.)
- Onion (.25 of 1)
- Ground beef (.66 lb.)
- Chopped cilantro (2 tbsp.)
- Red bell pepper (1)
- Fresh ginger (1 tsp.)
- Cumin (2 tsp.)
- Garlic cloves (4)
- Pepper and salt (as preferred)
- Large cabbage leaves (8)

Directions for Preparation:
1. Dice the bell pepper, onion, ginger, and garlic.
2. Warm a frying pan and pour some oil.
3. Sauté the peppers, onions, and ground beef using medium heat.
4. When done, add the black pepper, salt, cumin, ginger, cilantro, and garlic.
5. Scoop the mixture onto each leaf, fold, and serve.

Steak Pinwheels

Serving Yields Provided: 6
Macro Counts - Each Serving:
- Net Carbs: 2 g
- Total Fats: 19.5 g
- Protein: 54.5 g
- Calories: 414

Ingredients Needed:
- Flank steak (2 lb.)
- Mozzarella cheese (8 oz. pkg.)
- Spinach (about 1.75 cups, 1 bunch)

Directions for Preparation:
1. Warm the oven to 350° Fahrenheit.
2. Slice the steak into six portions, and remove all of the "hard" fat. Beat it thin with a mallet.
3. Shred the cheese using a food processor and sprinkle the steak. Roll it up and tie with a piece of cooking twine or a skewer.
4. Line the pan with the pinwheels and place on a layer of spinach. Bake until done (25 min.).

Stuffed Mushrooms

Serving Yields Provided: 4
Macro Counts - Each Serving:
- Net Carbs: 3 g Total Fats: 22 g
- Protein: 5 g Calories: 124

Ingredients Needed:
- Portobello mushrooms (4)
- Olive oil (2 tbsp.)
- Blue cheese (1 cup)
- Fresh thyme (1 pinch)
- Salt (as desired)

Directions for Preparation:
1. Warm the oven to 350° Fahrenheit.
2. Cut the stems from the mushrooms and chop them to bits.
3. Mix with the thyme, salt, and crumbled blue cheese and stuff the mushrooms.
4. Spritz with some of the oil.
5. Bake for 15 to 20 minutes. Serve as a delicious snack or side dish.

Sweet Snacks

Cinnamon Vanilla Protein Bites

Serving Yields Provided: 18–20 bites
Macro Counts - Each Serving:
- Net Carbs: 4 g
- Total Fats: 9 g
- Protein: 2 g
- Calories: 112

Ingredients Needed:
- Quick oats (.75 cup)
- Nut butter of choice (.25–.33 cup)
- Cinnamon (1 tbsp.)
- Pure maple syrup (.25–.33 cup)
- Vanilla protein powder (.25 cup)
- Almond meal (.5 cup)
- Vanilla extract (.5–1 tsp.)
- *Also Needed:* Food processor

Directions for Preparation:
1. Line a cookie tin with a layer of parchment paper.
2. Grind the oats with the processor and add to a mixing container. Combine the cinnamon, protein

powder, almond meal, and nut butter.

3. Mix in the syrup and vanilla. Using your hands, mix and roll them into small balls.
4. Freeze for 20 to 30 minutes.
5. Store in a Ziploc-type bag with the cinnamon and vanilla protein mixture.

Peanut Butter Protein Bars

Serving Yields Provided: 12 bars
Macro Counts - Each Serving:
- Net Carbs: 3 g
- Total Fats: 14 g
- Protein: 7 g
- Calories: 172

Ingredients Needed:
- Keto-friendly chunky peanut butter (1 cup)
- Egg whites (2)
- Almonds (.5 cup)
- Cashews (.5 cup)
- Almond meal (1.5 cups)

Directions for Preparation:
1. Warm up the oven ahead of time to 350° Fahrenheit.
2. Combine all of the fixings and add to the prepared dish.
3. Bake for 15 minutes.
4. Cut into 12 pieces once they're cool.
5. Store in the fridge to keep them fresh.

Chapter 31:

Dessert Favorites

Almond & Coconut Cake

Serving Yields Provided: 8
Macro Counts - Each Serving:
- Net Carbs: 3 g
- Total Fats: 23g
- Protein: 5 g
- Calories: 236

Dry Ingredients Needed:
- Almond flour (1 cup)
- Truvia (.33 cup)
- Baking powder (1 tsp.)
- Unsweetened shredded coconut (.5 cup)
- Apple pie spice (1 tsp.)

Wet Ingredients Needed:
- Melted butter (.25 cup)
- Lightly whisked eggs (2)
- Heavy whipping cream (.5 cup)

Directions for Preparation:
1. Combine all of the dry ingredients, and add each of the wet ingredients, one at a time. Empty the batter into the pan, and cover with foil.
2. Empty the water into the Kitchen robot, and place the steamer rack inside.
3. Set the timer 40 minutes using the high-pressure setting. Release the pressure naturally for 10 minutes, and then quick-release it.
4. Remove the pan, and let it cool for 15 to 20 minutes.
5. Flip it over onto a platter and garnish as desired (count the carbs).

6. It is very important to cool the cake completely before you add the toppings.

Brownie Mug Cake – Kitchen robot

Serving Yields Provided: 1
Macro Counts - Each Serving:
- Net Carbs: 1.3 g
- Protein: 9 g
- Total Fats: 12 g
- Calories: 143

Ingredients Needed:
- Whisked egg (1)
- Almond flour (.25 cup)
- Baking powder (.25 tsp.)
- Vanilla extract (.25 tsp.)
- Cacao powder (1.5 tbsp.)
- Cinnamon powder (1 tsp.)
- Stevia powder (2 tbsp.)
- Salt (1 pinch)

Directions for Preparation:
1. Pour one cup of water and the trivet or steam rack into the Kitchen robot.
2. Mix all of the fixings until well-combined, and pour it into a mug.
3. Cover with a piece of foil and place on the rack.
4. Secure the top.
5. Set the timer for 10 minutes using the "steam" button. Naturally, release the pressure (10 min.).
6. Cool for a minute and enjoy.

Cheesecake Pudding

Serving Yields Provided: 4
Macro Counts - Each Serving:
- Net Carbs: 5 g
- Total Fats: 36 g
- Protein: 5 g
- Calories: 356

Ingredients Needed:
- Cream cheese or Neufchatel cheese (1 block)
- Heavy whipping cream (.5 cup)
- Lemon juice (1 tsp.)
- Sour cream (.5 cup)
- Liquid stevia (20 drops)
- Vanilla extract (1 tsp.)

Directions for Preparation:
1. Microwave the cream cheese for 30 seconds, or leave it on the counter to soften for a few minutes before using.
2. Whip the sour cream and whipping cream together with the mixer until soft peaks form. Combine with the rest of the fixings and whip until fluffy.
3. Portion it into four dishes to chill. Place a layer of the wrap over the dish and store in the fridge.
4. When ready to eat, garnish with some berries if you like. If you add berries, make sure to add the carbs to the count.

Chocolate Chip Cookie Cheesecake Bars

Serving Yields Provided: 20
Macro Counts - Each Serving:
- Net Carbs: 5 g
- Protein: 5 g
- Total Fats: 25 g
- Calories: 280

Ingredients Needed - Cookies Crust:
- Almond flour (2 cups) - Shredded coconut (1 cup)
- Salt (.25 tsp.) - Swerve Sweetener (.5 cup)
- Baking powder (1.5 tsp.)
- Softened butter (.5 cup)
- Coconut sugar or more Swerve (2 tbsp.)
- Room temperature egg (1 large)
- Vanilla extract (.75 tsp.)
- Sugar-free chocolate chips (.5 cup)

Ingredients Needed - Cheesecake Filling:
- Large egg (1) - Cream cheese, softened (12 oz.)
- Powdered swerve (.33 cup)
- Whipping cream (.25 cup) - Vanilla extract (.5 tsp.)
- *Also Needed*: 9-inch square baking pan

Directions for Preparation - The Crust:
1. Warm the oven to 325° Fahrenheit.
2. Generously grease the pan.
3. Whisk the baking powder with the shredded coconut, almond flour, and salt in the mixing bowl.
4. In another container, beat the swerve with butter and coconut sugar. Whisk the vanilla and egg. Combine it with the flour mixture, and stir in the chocolate chips.
5. Press about 2/3 of the crust dough into the greased pan.
6. Bake for 10 to 12 minutes.
7. Take the tray out of the oven. Cool before adding the filling.

Directions for Preparation - The Filling:
1. Use a wooden spoon to blend the cheese with the sweetener and whipping cream until combined.

2. Whisk the vanilla extract and egg until smooth. Pour over the cooled crust.

3. Use the remainder of the cookie crust mixture to crumble over the top of the filling. Press gently to adhere.

4. Bake until the crust is nicely browned or for about 25 minutes. It will have just a little "jiggle" in the center. Transfer from the oven to cool completely.

5. Chill for at least 1 hour until set.

Chocolate-Filled Peanut Butter Cookies

Serving Yields Provided: 20
Macro Counts - Each Serving:
- Net Carbs: 2.7 g
- Protein: 4.5 g
- Total Fats: 14 g
- Calories: 150

Ingredients Needed:
- Almond flour (2.5 cups)
- Baking powder (1.5 tsp.)
- Salt (.5 tsp.)
- Peanut butter (.5 cup)
- Coconut oil (.25 cup)
- Erythritol (.25 cup)
- Maple syrup (3 tbsp.)
- Dark chocolate bars (2-3)
- Vanilla extract (1 tbsp.)

Directions for Preparation:
1. Prepare the cookie pan with a baking paper.
2. Warm the oven to reach 350° Fahrenheit.
3. Whisk each of the wet fixings together and mix with the dry ingredients.
4. Mix well and store in the refrigerator for 20 to 30 minutes.
5. Break the bars into small squares. Press them until they are flat.

6. Add one to two pieces of chocolate and seal them into the ball.
7. Arrange them on the cookie sheet.
8. Bake for about 15 minutes.

Chocolate Mini Cakes

Serving Yields Provided: 2
Macro Counts - Each Serving:
- Net Carbs: 9 g
- Total Fats: 12 g
- Protein: 15 g
- Calories: 193

Ingredients Needed:
- Large eggs (2)
- Splenda/your favorite sweetener (2 tbsp.)
- Baking cocoa (.25 cup)
- Heavy cream (2 tbsp.)
- Baking powder (.5 tsp.)
- Vanilla extract (1 tsp.)
- Water (1 cup)

Directions for Preparation:
1. Add the water and trivet into the Kitchen robot.
2. Combine all of the dry ingredients and mix well.
3. Mix in another dish, and blend in the rest of the ingredients (eggs, cream, vanilla extract).
4. Spray the ramekins with oil, and fill each one halfway with the mixture. Carefully add them to the cooker and secure the lid.
5. Prepare for 9 minutes using the high-pressure setting.
6. Quick-release the pressure, and transfer the ramekins to a plate to cool.
7. Make sure they are cool before adding toppings, or you can serve hot right out of the ramekins.

Coconut-Almond Bars – Kitchen robot

Serving Yields Provided: 6
Macro Counts - Each Serving:
- Net Carbs: 2 g Total Fats: 25 g
- Protein: 5 g Calories: 253

Ingredients Needed:
- Coconut oil (.5 cup)
- Almond flour (1.25 cups)
- Coconut flour (.25 cup
- Eggs (2)
- Sugar substitute (3 tbsp.)
- Almond butter (2 tbsp.)
- Salt (.25 tsp.)
- Water (1 cup)
- Vanilla extract (1 tsp.)

Also Needed:
- Trivet for the Cooker & Baking pan to fit inside
- Food processor

Directions for Preparation:
1. Line the pan that fits in the cooker with the baking paper.
2. Combine all of the fixings in the food processor and add to the pan.
3. Empty the water into the Kitchen robot with the steamer rack. Arrange the pan in the cooker and secure the lid.
4. Set the timer for 15 minutes.
5. Natural-release the pressure and chill the pan until its room temperature.
6. Slice into six bars.

Creamy Lime Pie

Serving Yields Provided: 8
Macro Counts - Each Serving:
- Net Carbs: 4.2 g Protein: 7 g
- Total Fats: 38.6 g Calories: 386

Ingredients Needed:
- Almond flour (1.5 cups)
- Erythritol (divided, .5 cup)
- Salt (.5 tsp.)
- Melted butter (.25 cup)
- Heavy cream (1 cup)
- Egg yolks (4)
- Freshly squeezed key lime juice (.33 cup)
- Lime zest (1 tbsp.)
- Cubed cold butter (.25 cup)
- Vanilla extract (1 tsp.)
- Xanthan gum (.25 tsp.)
- Sour cream (1 cup)
- Cream cheese (.5 cup)

Directions for Preparation:
1. Warm the oven to 350° Fahrenheit.
2. Melt the butter in a pan.
3. Mix the salt, half or .25 cup of erythritol, and the almond flour. Slowly add the butter. Blend and press into a pie platter.
4. Bake for 15 minutes. Remove when it's lightly browned. Let it cool.
5. In another saucepan, combine the egg yolks, heavy cream, and the rest of the erythritol, lime zest, and juice.
6. Simmer using medium heat for 7 to 10 minutes or until it starts to thicken.
7. Take the pan from the heat, and add the xanthan gum, vanilla extract, cold butter, cream cheese, and sour cream. Whisk until smooth.
8. Scoop into the cooled pie shell. Cover and place in the fridge.
9. You can serve after 4 hours, but it is better if you wait overnight to enjoy the delicious treat.

5-Minute Peanut Butter Mousse

Serving Yields Provided: 4
Macro Counts - Each Serving:
- Net Carbs: 3 g Total Fats: 26.5 g
- Protein: 5.9 g
- Calories: 301

Ingredients Needed:

- Heavy whipping cream, more if needed to thin the mixture (.5 cup)
- Cream cheese, softened (4 oz.)
- Natural peanut butter, no sugar added (.25 cup)
- Powdered Swerve Sweetener (.25 cup)
- Vanilla extract (.5 tsp.)

Directions for Preparation:

1. Whisk or whip the cream until it holds stiff peaks. Set aside.
2. In another medium bowl, beat together the cream cheese and peanut butter until smooth and creamy. Add the sweetener and vanilla. If your peanut butter is unsalted, add a pinch of salt as well. Beat until smooth.
3. If your mixture is very thick, add about 2 tbsp heavy cream to lighten it. Beat it again until combined.
4. Gently fold in the whipped cream until no streaks remain. Spoon or pipe into dessert glasses.

Keto Magic Bars

Serving Yields Provided: 16
Macro Counts - Each Serving:
- Net Carbs: 4.5 g
- Total Fats: 12.4 g
- Protein: 1.8 g
- Calories: 132

Ingredients Needed:

- Almond flour (1.5 cups)
- Sweetener of choice, or stevia equivalent (2 tbsp.)
- Melted coconut oil (3 tbsp.)
- Salt (.25 tsp.)
- Mini chocolate chips or sugar-free chocolate chips (.75 cup)
- Full-fat shredded coconut (.66 cup)
- Full-fat canned coconut milk (1.25 cup)

- *Optional:* Walnuts (.25 cup)
- *Optional*: Cocoa powder (2 tbsp.)
- *Also Needed*: 8-inch baking pan

Directions for Preparation:

1. Finely chop the walnuts. Prepare the pan with a layer of parchment baking paper.
2. Toss the salt, sweetener, almond flour, and oil together in the mixing bowl.
3. Press the mixture into the papered pan.
4. Toss the coconut, chips of chocolate, and nuts over the top.
5. Stir the cocoa with the coconut milk. Pour this evenly over the top.
6. Bake for 33 minutes.
7. Transfer the bars from the oven.
8. Let them cool for about 15 minutes to firm up.
9. Slice into bars, wiping the knife after each cut.

No-Bake Cheesecake

Serving Yields Provided: 6
Macro Counts - Each Serving:
- Net Carbs: 5 g
- Total Fats: 25 g
- Protein: 7 g
- Calories: 247

Ingredients Needed - The Crust:

- Almond flour (2 tbsp.)
- Melted coconut oil (2 tbsp.)
- Swerve Confectioners or equivalent (2 tbsp.)
- Crushed salted almonds (2 tbsp.)

Ingredients Needed - The Filling:

- Gelatin (1 tsp.)
- Swerve confectioners or equivalent (.25 cup)
- Cream cheese (16 oz. pkg.)
- Unsweetened almond milk (.5 cup)
- Vanilla extract (1 tsp.)

Directions for Preparation:

1. Prepare the crust by combining all of the fixings under the crust section. Place one heaping tablespoon into the bottom of the dessert cups. Press the mixture down and set aside.
2. Prepare the filling. Mix the sweetener and gelatin. Pour in the milk and stir (5 min.). Whip the vanilla beans and cream cheese with a mixer using the medium setting until creamy. Add the gelatin mixture slowly until well-incorporated.
3. Pour the mixture over the crust of each cup. Chill for 3 hours, minimum.

No-Bake Chocolate Fudge Haystacks

Serving Yields Provided: 12
Macro Counts - Each Serving:
- Net Carbs: 1.5 g
- Total Fats: 18 g
- Protein: 2 g
- Calories: 172

Ingredients Needed:
- Softened cream cheese (4 oz.)
- Erythritol sweetener (.75 cup)
- Softened unsalted butter (.5 cup)
- Unsweetened cocoa powder (.25 cup)
- Coarse sea salt (.125 tsp.)
- Unsweetened desiccated/shredded coconut (1 cup)
- Sugar-free vanilla extract (1 tsp.)
- Chopped walnuts (.33 cups)

Directions for Preparation:
1. Blend the cocoa powder, sweetener, cheese, and butter.
2. Stir in the walnuts, coconut, salt, and vanilla extract.

3. Scoop out 1-inch balls to make haystacks. Chill for approximately 30 minutes or longer.
4. Store in the refrigerator or freezer for best results.

Peanut Butter Fudge

Serving Yields Provided: 20
Macro Counts - Each Serving:
- Net Carbs: 6 g
- Total Fats: 11 g
- Protein: 4 g
- Calories: 135

Ingredients Needed:
- Coconut oil (3 tbsp.)
- Smooth peanut butter, keto-friendly (12 oz.)
- Coconut cream (4 tbsp.)
- Maple syrup (4 tbsp.)
- Salt (1 pinch)

Directions for Preparation:
1. Prepare a baking sheet with a layer of parchment paper.
2. Melt the syrup and coconut oil using the medium heat setting on the stovetop.
3. Stir in the salt, coconut cream, and peanut butter. Pour the mixture into the prepared dish and chill in the fridge for at least 1 hour.
4. Slice into pieces and store or serve.

Pumpkin Caramel Bundt Cake

Serving Yields Provided: 16
Macro Counts - Each Serving:
- Net Carbs: 5 g
- Total Fats: 16.5 g
- Protein: 8 g
- Calories: 212

Ingredients Needed - The Cake:
- Almond flour (2.5 cups)

- Coconut flour (.5 cup)
- Swerve sweetener (.66 cup)
- Baking powder (1 tbsp.)
- Unflavored whey protein powder (.33 cup)
- Cinnamon (2 tsp.)
- Ginger (1 tsp.) - Salt (.5 tsp.)
- Cloves (.25 tsp.)
- Pumpkin puree (1.5 cups)
- Large eggs (4)
- Melted butter (.25 cup)
- Water (.5 to .66 cup)
- Vanilla extract (1 tsp.)

Ingredients Needed - The Glaze:
- Butter (.25 cup)
- Molasses for color and flavor (1 tsp.)
- Powdered Swerve sweetener (.5 cup)
- Caramel flavor (.5 tsp.)
- Whipping cream (2 tbsp.)

Directions for Preparation - Cake Preparation:
1. Warm up the oven to 325° Fahrenheit.
2. Grease the pan well. Whisk the coconut flour, almond flour, sweetener, protein powder, salt, baking powder, cloves, and ginger in the mixing bowl.
3. Fold in the eggs, pumpkin puree, 1/2 cup water, butter, and vanilla extract. Add small amounts of water as needed for a thick consistency.
4. Empty the batter into the greased pan.
5. Bake 55 to 60 minutes. Test for doneness.
6. Remove and let cool 15 minutes. Place onto the rack to cool.

Directions for Preparation - The Glaze:
1. In the pan, using low heat, melt butter with molasses or yacon syrup. Stir it until smooth.

2. Take the pan off the burner and stir in powdered sweetener, caramel extract, and whipping cream. Drizzle over the cooled cake. It's also grain-free.

Raspberry Fudge

Serving Yields Provided: 12
Macro Counts - Each Serving:
- Net Carbs: 4.4 g Protein: 2.6 g
- Total Fats: 25.3 g Calories: 242

Ingredients Needed:
- Cream cheese (16 oz.)
- Butter (1 cup)
- Heavy cream (2 tbsp.)
- White sugar substitute (.25 cup)
- Unsweetened cocoa powder (6 tbsp.)
- Vanilla extract (2 tsp.)
- Raspberry extract (1 tsp.)
- Chopped walnuts (.33 cup)

Directions for Preparation:
1. Take the cream cheese and butter out of the fridge ahead of time until it is cooled to room temperature.
2. Mix the cream cheese and butter in a mixing bowl with the mixer.
3. When smooth, mix with the rest of the fixings until well-incorporated.
4. Microwave it using the high setting for 30 seconds. Blend it with the mixer again until smooth.
5. Empty the mixture into the prepared pan (1-inch layer). Cover it and chill for at least 2 hours in the fridge.
6. Slice into 12 portions.
7. Serve or store in the fridge.

Raspberry Ice Cream

Serving Yields Provided: 5
Macro Counts - Each Serving - .5 cup each::
- Net Carbs: 3 g Protein: 1 g
- Total Fats: 16 g Calories: 183

Ingredients Needed:

- Heavy cream (or coconut cream (1 cup)
- Frozen raspberries (2 cups)
- Powdered erythritol or any sweetener, to taste (.33 cup)

Directions for Preparation:

1. Pour the cream into a blender. Blend until stiff peaks form (you can also use a hand mixer if your blender isn't powerful enough to whip the cream).
2. Add the frozen raspberries and sweetener to the blender. Puree until incorporated. Adjust the sweetener to taste, and puree it again if needed.
3. *Note:* If you prefer firmer ice cream; you can run the mixture through an ice cream maker, or place it in the freezer to firm up.
4. If you're using the freezer, stir every 30–60 minutes for the first couple hours to break up any ice crystals.

Sugar-Free Fudgesicles

Serving Yields Provided: 8
Macro Counts - Each Serving:
- Net Carbs: 1.6 g
- Protein: 1.44 g
- Total Fats: 11.2 g
- Calories: 118

Ingredients Needed:

- Heavy cream (1 cup)
- Almond or cashew milk unsweetened (1 cup)
- Unsweetened cocoa powder (.33 cup)
- Swerve Sweetener (.33 cup)
- Vanilla extract or peppermint extract (1 tsp.)
- Xanthan gum (.25 tsp.)
- *Also Needed:* Wooden sticks

Directions for Preparation:

1. Whisk the swerve, cream, milk, and cocoa powder in a saucepan using the medium-high heat setting. Cook for 1 minute after it starts to boil.
2. Transfer the pan from the burner, and add the flavoring.
3. Add the xanthan gum and whisk well.
4. Chill for a minimum of 10 minutes before pouring into the molds.
5. Freeze for at least another hour. Push the popsicle sticks into the mixture, but not all the way, and then return the mold to the freezer.
6. When you're ready to enjoy it, pour a bit of hot water over the mold to release the popsicles.

Vanilla Shortbread Cookies

Serving Yields Provided: 16
Macro Counts - Each Serving:
- Net Carbs: 1 g
- Total Fats: 12 g
- Protein: 3 g
- Calories: 126

Ingredients Needed:

- Almond flour (2 cups)
- Erythritol (.33 cup)
- Salt (1 pinch)
- Egg (1 large)
- Softened unsalted butter (.5 cup)
- Vanilla extract (1 tsp.)

Directions for Preparation:

1. Warm the oven to reach 300° Fahrenheit.
2. Combine the almond flour with the salt, erythritol, salt, and vanilla extract.
3. Toss in the butter and rub into the dry ingredients until fully mixed.
4. Fold in the whisked egg.
5. Roll tablespoon-sized pieces of the mixture into balls.

6. Press onto a lined cookie sheet. Leave a gap between the cookies.
7. Bake until the edges are browned (for 15 to 25 min.).
8. The cookies will firm up as they cool. Leave to cool before storing in an airtight jar.
9. *Note*: It's recommended to use gloves to prevent the mixture from sticking to your hands.

Vanilla Sour Cream Cupcake

Serving Yields Provided: 12
Macro Counts - Each Serving:
- Net Carbs: 2 g
- Protein: 4 g
- Total Fats: 11 g
- Calories: 128

Ingredients Needed:
- Butter (4 tbsp.)
- Swerve or your favorite sweetener (1.5 cups)
- Eggs (4)
- Vanilla (1 tsp.)
- Sour cream (.25 cup)
- Almond flour (1 cup)
- Coconut flour (.25 cup)
- Baking powder (1 tsp.)
- Salt (.25 tsp.)
- *Also Needed*: 12-count muffin tin

Directions for Preparation:
1. Heat the oven to reach 350° Fahrenheit. Prepare the muffin cups with paper liners.
2. Use an electric mixer to cream the butter and sweetener until creamy smooth. Fold in the vanilla and sour cream. Continue mixing, adding the rest of the eggs, one at a time.
3. Stir in both of the flour options, salt, and baking powder. Blend well.
4. Pour the batter into the cups.
5. Bake for 20–30 minutes until they are golden brown.

6. Cool completely and store in the fridge.

Zucchini Chocolate Cake

Serving Yields Provided: 10
Macro Counts - Each Serving:
- Net Carbs: 7.4 g
- Protein: 10.1 g
- Total Fats: 26.5 g
- Calories: 306

Ingredients Needed:
- Almond flour (3 cups)
- Baking soda (1 tsp.)
- Coconut flour (.25 cup)
- Cacao powder (.5 cup)
- Eggs (4)
- Vanilla extract (3 tsp.)
- Apple cider vinegar (1 tbsp.)
- Melted cacao butter (.25 cup)
- Coconut cream (.75 cup)
- Grated zucchini (2 cups)
- Non-GMO erythritol, birch xylitol, or a blend such as Lakanto (6 tbsp.)
- Salt (1 pinch)

Directions for Preparation:
1. Heat the oven in advance until it reaches 350° Fahrenheit.
2. Prepare the pan with baking paper or a spritz of coconut oil or ghee.
3. Combine the dry components and toss with the rest fixings until combined.
4. Dump the batter into the cake tin.
5. Bake it until it is no longer wobbly in the middle (for 30 to 40 min.). Test the cake for doneness with a cake tester or a sharp knife.
6. Cool it completely and serve plain or with whipped coconut cream, berries, or a simple chocolate glaze.

Chapter 32:

21-Day Special Meal Plan for Busy People

Each of these recipes has the net carbs per serving posted. You will see how flexible the plan is when you look at how easy it is to use the recipes in this cookbook for 21 full days, including three meals, snacks, and desserts.

The meals are planned, so you still have flexibility in your eating patterns with extra carbs to use as desired. Even on the strictest diet plan, most of these recipes should be just what the doctor ordered. You have plenty of extra choices, so just enjoy.

Calculate how many carbs you are allowed each day, and add some healthy snacks or sides to the carb count. It's all up to you; just track everything.

Day 1:

Breakfast: Blueberry Flaxseed Muffins: 8.78 grams
Lunch: Egg Salad: 1.4 grams
Dinner: Mongolian Beef: 1.99 grams
Snack or Dessert: Stuffed Mushrooms: 3 grams

Day 2:

Breakfast: Eggs & Sausage Breakfast Sandwich: 6 grams
Lunch: Jalapeno Popper Chicken Salad: 0 grams
Dinner: Stuffed Pork Tenderloin on the Grill: 3 grams
Snack or Dessert: Creamy Lime Pie: 4.2 grams

Day 3:

Breakfast: Pulled Pork Hash: 8 grams
Lunch: Simple Red Cabbage Salad: 0.2 grams
Dinner: BBQ Flank Steak: 1 gram
Snack or Dessert: Pumpkin Caramel Bundt Cake: 5 grams

Day 4:

Breakfast: Smoothie in a Bowl: 4 grams
Lunch: Sloppy Joes – Vegan: 8.9 grams
Dinner: Chicken BBQ Zucchini Boats: 9 grams
Snack or Dessert: Vanilla Shortbread Cookies: 1 gram

Day 5:

Breakfast: Green Buttered Eggs: 2.5 grams
Lunch: Chicken BLT Salad: 4 grams
Dinner: Hamburger Stroganoff: 6 grams
Snack or Dessert: Chocolate Chip Cookie Cheesecake Bars: 5 grams

Day 6:

Breakfast: Cinnamon Raisin Bagels: 6 grams
Lunch: Chicken 'Zoodle' Soup: 4 grams
Dinner: Carnitas – Crockpot: 4 grams
Snack or Dessert: Peanut Butter Fudge: 6 grams

Day 7:

Breakfast: Porridge: 5.4 grams
Lunch: Avocado & Salmon Omelet Wrap: 5.8 grams
Dinner: Barbacoa Beef – Kitchen robot: 2 grams
Snack or Dessert: Raspberry Ice Cream: 3 grams

Day 8:

Breakfast: Belgian Style Waffles: 3 grams
Lunch: Vegetarian Club Salad: 5 grams
Dinner: Baked Tilapia With Cherry Tomatoes: 4 grams
Snack or Dessert: Vanilla Sour Cream Cupcake: 2 grams

Day 9:

Breakfast: Creamy Basil Baked Sausage: 4 grams
Lunch: Warm Peach Scallops Salad: 7 grams
Dinner: Nacho Skillet Steak: 6 grams
Snack or Dessert: Brownie Mug Cake – Kitchen robot: 1.3 grams

Day 10:

Breakfast: Almond Coconut Egg Wraps: 3 grams
Lunch: Chicken Chowder – Crockpot: 7.5 grams

Dinner: Lemon Shrimp: 2.5 grams & Arancini – 5-Cheese Bacon & Cauliflower Bites: 5.4 grams
Snack or Dessert: Sugar-Free Fudgesicles: 1.6 grams

Day 11:

Breakfast: Biscuits & Gravy: 2 grams
Lunch: Greek Salad: 8 grams
Dinner: Cheeseburger Calzones: 3 grams
Snack or Dessert: Keto Magic Bars: 4.5 grams

Day 12:

Breakfast: Pesto Scrambled Eggs: 2.6 grams
Lunch: Alfredo Shrimp: 6.5 grams
Dinner: Chicken & Asparagus: 4 grams
Snack or Dessert: Cheesecake Pudding: 5 grams

Day 13:

Breakfast: Spinach Quiche: 0 grams
Lunch: Chicken, Feta, & Kiwi Salad: 13 grams
Dinner: Bacon Cheeseburger: 0.8 grams
Snack or Dessert: Raspberry Fudge: 4.4 grams

Day 14:

Breakfast: Keto Hot Cross Buns: 2.1 grams
Lunch: Caprese Salad: 4.6 grams
Dinner: Roasted Chicken & Tomatoes: 5 grams
Snack or Dessert: Zucchini Chocolate Cake: 7.4 grams

Day 15:

Breakfast: Almost McGriddle Casserole: 3 grams
Lunch: No-Cook Chilled Avocado & Mint Soup: 4 grams
Dinner: Enchilada: 7 grams
Snack or Dessert: 5-Minute Peanut Butter Mousse: 3 grams

Day 16:

Breakfast: Chocolate Loaf: 2.32 grams
Lunch: Jar Salad with Tempeh – Vegan: 4 grams
Dinner: Slow-Cooked Kalua Pork & Cabbage: 4 grams
Snack or Dessert: Chocolate-Filled Peanut Butter Cookies: 2.7 grams

Day 17:

Breakfast: Bacon Hash: 9 grams
Lunch: Creamy Chicken Soup: 2 grams

Dinner: Slow-Cooked London Broil: 2.5 grams
Snack or Dessert: Almond & Coconut Cake: 3 grams

Day 18:

Breakfast: Cocoa Waffles: 3.4 grams
Lunch: Lobster Salad: 2 grams
Dinner: Parmesan Crusted Pork Chops: 3 grams
Snack or Dessert: Coconut Almond Bars – Kitchen robot: 2 grams

Day 19:

Breakfast: Pumpkin Pancakes: 4 grams
Lunch: Broccoli Curry Soup: 4.8 grams
Dinner: Crack Slaw – Pork Egg Roll in a Bowl: 5.5 grams
Snack or Dessert: No-Bake Chocolate Fudge Haystacks: 1.5 grams

Day 20:

Breakfast: Almonds & Chips Breakfast Cereal: 3 grams
Lunch: Fish Cakes: 0.6 grams & Chinese Sauce Fried Rice: 4.3 grams

Dinner: Sesame Chicken Egg Roll in a Bowl: 3.3 grams
Snack or Dessert: Cinnamon Vanilla Protein Bites: 4 grams

Day 21:

Breakfast: Bagels & Cheese: 8 grams
Lunch: Tuna Salad & Chives: 1 gram
Dinner: BBQ Pork Loin: 3 grams
Snack or Dessert: Chocolate Mini Cakes: 9 grams

Chapter 33:

Tips & Tricks to Control Hunger & Avoid Mistakes

How to Maintain Fat Loss

Remain Consistent During Fasting: Regardless of the type of weight loss that you ultimately choose to pursue, it's essential to pick one and stick with it. Attempting an intermittent fast for a few days using the keto diet plan before switching to another program, such as the Paleo diet, before trying out a low-carb approach will only cause your body to become confused. It will hold on to every possible calorie until it figures out what the changes mean.

Remember, fasting regularly and consistently is the surest way to see any of its benefits. Only after your body has time to adjust to your new routine will it then be able to adapt appropriately. It can begin to increase the number of positive enzymes and neural pathways to maximize weight loss using this method. Consider consistency of the "ace-in-the-hole" of proactive weight loss success.

Maintain Your Self-Control: Intermittent fasting only works if your body goes entirely without food for at least twelve hours; any caloric intake resets the cycle. As such, it is imperative to ensure that you maintain control of your bodily urges if you hope to see real results from this type of approach. Remember, fasting for at least twelve hours will only allow you to eat as you usually would or slightly more than an average meal. It doesn't give you free rein to eat everything in sight. Keeping your appetite in check is a strict requirement for success.

Maintain a Calorie Deficit: While this is true for any diet, it is even more true for intermittent fasting since it can be so easy to overeat in such a way that it negates any benefits you might have felt. Remember, you need to burn 3,500 calories on average weekly to lose one pound each week.

Avoid Junk Food: While intermittent fasting means that you will likely have a little extra caloric room in your diet for junk food if you so choose, trying to eat poorly while intermittent fasting will only lead to failure. While you may technically be able to spare the calories, spending the ones you do have on things that won't stick to your ribs for the long haul is a recipe for disaster. Focus on foods that are high in protein and healthy fats. You will feel full and energetic for more prolonged periods every time. You only have so much time you can eat each day, so make it count.

Take It Slow: If you have never gone more than a few hours without eating, then it's a good idea to start slowly. You can go hours without eating and then build up your tolerance from there. It is important to go slow, so if you experience lots of failures early on, it can be more challenging to convince your brain to get into a pro-fasting mindset in the long term. Once you begin to see real weight loss results, you will notice that it will become easier to persevere; all you have to do is make it to that point, and things will begin to fall into place.

Be Aware Of Your Body's Response: While you will want to monitor how your body is reacting to the intermittent fasting process as long as you are regularly withholding calories, this is especially important during the first month while your body is transitioning to a new way of receiving calories. While you may feel faint, lightheaded, shaky, irritable, angry, or weak for up to a month while fasting, symptoms that persist indefinitely are a sign that something ultimately isn't right. It is essential to be in touch with your body enough to know when it's time to consult a health care professional.

Drink Tons of Water: This doesn't mean merely stay hydrated, which is good advice, regardless. It means you should drink at least a gallon of water each day. It will help you feel full and also ensure your body continues processing toxins normally, even if it is holding onto all of its fat because of the transition that is occurring. This is a good exercise for most people anyway, as roughly 40 percent of adults are in a mild state of dehydration. If thirst remains untreated for long enough, it starts manifesting itself as hunger, so staying hydrated will keep you feeling full longer in two ways. *Plan On Staying Busy:* While this is a good suggestion in general when it comes to the final few hours of your fast, it's especially important during your transition period. Having nothing to do but sit around for several hours until you can eat again is a sure way to put your untrained body into a situation where it can't help but fail. Don't let this happen to you. Just ensure your fast will break after a period of constant mental activity, and you will find those last few hours going by much faster.

Get More Sleep & Less Stress: If you are a victim of sleep deprivation, you will understand how stressful everyday life is, even before you begin a diet plan. You may believe it's too late for you, but it isn't. Your diet plan will work, but you may need to make a few other adjustments. Chronic stress will increase your cortisol levels—the stress hormone. With that action, your hunger levels also rise. The result is that you eat more and put on weight. It's important to find ways to remove the stress, whether it is decluttering your home or taking a vacation.
Eliminate coffee or other forms of caffeine early in the afternoon, and don't consume alcohol for at least three hours before bedtime. Alcohol will also interfere with your quality of sleep, which is why you wake up feeling tired after an evening of nightclubs and boozing.

Recognize Your Cravings

Sugary Foods: Several things can trigger one's desire for sugar, but typically, phosphorous, and tryptophan are the culprits. Have some chicken, beef, lamb, liver, cheese, cauliflower, or broccoli.

Chocolate: The carbon, magnesium, and chromium levels are requesting a portion of spinach, nuts, and seeds, or some broccoli and cheese. It's important to make sure you keep a healthy count of sodium, potassium, and magnesium in your diet. It is suggested to consume a minimum of two teaspoons daily. However, if you crave chocolate, eat chocolate. You need to make sure you eat 75% or higher dark chocolate. Omit milk chocolate from the diet plan.

Fatty or Oily Foods: The levels of calcium and chloride need repair with some spinach, broccoli, cheese, or fish.

Carbs/Bread/Pasta: You need some nitrogen, which can be remedied by eating high-protein meat.

Eat Healthier Snacks During Your Eating Window

Stock your pantry with plenty of high-quality snacks that you can eat when your resistance is down. When you choose snack items, always be sure to select ones that are low in carbs, so your ketone levels will not be disrupted. If you have a busy lifestyle, pick some of the items in the following list, but always remember to count the carbs.

- *Pork Rinds:* Use these to replace chips and crackers. For example, try Pork Clouds, which has a higher quality but without a lot of the offensive oil content.

- *Pepperoni Slices:* Enjoy them with high-fat cheese products, but keep in mind that these are highly processed. Limit your intake of this, and search for hormone-free meat or organic food, if possible.

- *String Cheese:* Choose the full-fat version without additional fillers.

- *Laughing Cow Cheese Wheels:* Purchase full-fat versions and get *real* cheese when possible.

- *Iced Coffee*: Leave the sugar out of your coffee, and use only full-fat milk or cream. Add a bit of MCT oil powder, which can be purchased as chocolate, vanilla, or unflavored.

- *Stevia Sweetened Dark Chocolate*: If you are not using stevia, make sure it's a minimum of 80% or higher in cocoa content.

- *Cacao Nibs*: You can enjoy the same crunch when used as an alternative to chocolate chips.

- *Sugar-Free Jell-O or Popsicles*: You can purchase this ready-to-go, or you can make your own.

Be Sure the Plan Is for You—Avoid Mistakes

As with other things in your life, intermittent fasting may not be for you. You may need to avoid the restrictions if you are included in these categories:

- People with eating disorder histories

- If you are taking prescription medications, you can have issues on taking them on an empty stomach. If you have diabetes, Metformin may cause diarrhea or nausea. Iron supplements may also cause stomach discomfort. Aspirin may also cause an upset stomach or possible ulcers.

- Individuals with diabetes mellitus: type 1 or type 2

- Individuals who experience a drop in his/her blood sugar levels many times

- People who are underweight (BMI≤ 18.5), malnourished, or have other known nutrient deficiencies

- Pregnant women will need more nutrition for the unborn child.

- Nursing mothers will require more nutrients for the baby.

- Children under 18 need more nutrients to grow.

Other Intermittent Dieting Suggestions

If you have tried the 16/8 plan without success, try one of these options.
Skipping Meals: If you're interested in trying out the benefits of intermittent fasting for yourself, but you have an irregular schedule or are not sure if it is for you, then skipping a meal or two, now and then, maybe the type of intermittent fasting for you. As previously discussed, getting into a fasting routine is vital to see the maximum results for your effort, but that doesn't occasionally mean that fasting doesn't come with some benefits as well.

What's more, once you have tried skipping a meal now and then, you can see for yourself just how easy it is, which, in turn, can lead to more positive changes in the future. With so many intermittent fasting options available, the odds are good that one fits your schedule, so give it a try. What have you got to lose, except for a bunch of unessential pounds?

Alternate Day Diet: This form of intermittent fasting means you never have to go long without food if you don't wish to fast for an extended time. Every other day, you should eat regularly, and on the off-days, you merely consume one-fifth of the calories you usually intake on average days.

The average daily caloric consumption is between 2,000 and 2,500 calories, which means that the regular off-day varies between 400 and 500 calories. If you enjoy exercising every day, then this form of intermittent fasting may not be for you since you will have to limit your workouts on off-days severely.

When you first begin this technique of intermittent fasting, the easiest way to make it through the low-calorie days is by trying any the protein shakes listed. It is important to work back to "real" natural foods these days because they will always be healthier than the shakes.

This form of intermittent fasting is all about losing weight. Those who try it tend to average between two and three pounds lost per week. If you attempt the Alternate Day Diet, it is critical to eat regularly on your full-calorie days. Binging will not only negate any progress you've made, but it can also cause severe damage to your body if continued over time.

Crescendo Method: This is a method that is ranked as one method suitable for women since you can begin fasting without irritating your hormones or shocking any part of your body using this technique. This is one of the safest programs for women who utilize a fasting window of 12-16 hours. You can enjoy your meals for 8-12 hours. Space it out for a few days, such as Monday, Wednesday, and Friday. If you have failed other diets, this might be your answer. After a two-week period, add one more day of active fasting to your schedule.

Always Check Your Medications for Compatibility

It's important to inform your doctor about your weight loss program. He/she may prescribe some medicines that make you gain weight.

If you are taking insulin injections in high doses, your insulin can impede weight loss. By consuming fewer carbs, you are substantially reducing the requirement of insulin. Again, ask your healthcare professional before you make any changes.

If you are attempting to lose weight, be aware of other probable medications causing weight gain:

- Oral contraceptives
- Antidepressants
- Epilepsy drugs
- Blood pressure medications
- Allergy medicines
- Antibiotics

Know-How: Test for Ketosis Activity

Maintaining ketosis is an individual process, and you need to be sure you are achieving your goals. The levels of beta-hydroxybutyrate, acetone, and acetoacetate can be measured in your urine, breath, and blood.

You can use a *"Ketonix"* meter to measure your breath. You breathe into the meter. The results will be provided by a special coded color that will flash to show your levels of ketosis at that time.

Measure the ketones with a blood ketone meter. All it takes is a small drop of blood on a testing strip inserted into the meter. This process has been researched as an excellent indicator of your current ketosis levels. Unfortunately, the testing strips are expensive.

Test your urine for acetoacetate. The strip is dipped into the urine, which will change the color of the strip. The various shades of purple and pink indicate the levels of ketones. The darker the color on the testing strip, the higher the level of ketones. The major benefit of this is that they are inexpensive. The most effective time to test is early in the morning, after a ketogenic diet dinner, the evening before testing.

You should use one or more of these methods to indicate whether you need to adjust your intake of foods to remain in ketosis.

When you fast, the hormones in your body will change. The keto plan is similar to this process. You could achieve ketosis in just a couple of days once you have used up all your stored glycogen. It can take a month, a week, or just a few days. It all depends on which type of plan you choose. Your protein and carbohydrate intake will determine the time.

Conclusion

I hope you enjoyed every segment of *Intermittent Fasting*, from the first page to the end, and I hope you can now achieve your goals in weight loss or whatever they may be.

The next step is to gather your essential shopping list and knowledge on the ketogenic diet to travel to the supermarket.

- Prepare the food list consisting of your favorite spices and other products to convert your pantry to keto.

- Begin using your new diet plan, remembering that you can adjust the menu plan using the carbohydrate limitations set for each day. Keep your intake of carbs low.

- Prepare a food journal, and familiarize yourself with an online app to remain in ketosis with ease. You have all of the tools to be successful, but you still need to understand how to test yourself to ensure that you are in ketosis. Your individual progress can be tested using several items to ensure you remain in a ketogenic state. They include testing your breath, blood, or urine.

There is no time like the present to gather your lists of goods needed to begin your ketogenic way of living. Begin with your food and preparation items, and before you know it, you will be stocking your freezer to the brim with all the delicious keto foods your body is craving.

If you find yourself feeling excessively hungry in the early morning hours, the first thing you should keep in mind is that much of this hunger is actually mental, rather than physical. After you have finished the transition, you should notice it much less often. With that being said, it's important to start each day by drinking a liter of water. If you still feel hungry, consider ending your previous day's meal with extra protein and healthy fats which should stick with you through the morning.

Above all, reward yourself. After you have started losing weight, it is important to have a bit of fun. However, you should make sure that it is not a food-related treat. Treat yourself to a massage, or buy a new pair of jeans to show off your loss. Take the family for a game of putt-putt or enjoy a special spa treatment. You deserve it.

While you are considering your reward, why not have a delicious cup of coffee?
This Bulletproof Coffee is for one serving with zero carbs. It has 51 total fats, 1 protein, and 320 calories.

Ingredients Needed:
- MCT oil powder (2 tbsp.)
- Ghee or butter (2 tbsp.)
- Hot coffee (1.5 cups)

Directions for Preparation:
1. Empty the hot coffee into your blender.
2. Pour in the powder and butter. Blend until frothy.
3. Enjoy using a large mug.

Finally, if you found this book useful in any way, a review on Amazon is always appreciated!

Thank you for reading this book!

I hope it will help you and your life!

This is a little present for you.

Click here to download your meal plan to save it on your phone or to print it and keep in your kitchen, to remember always what to eat.

https://www.mediafire.com/file/5onunbarz4wd014/Meal_Plan.pdf/file

PS: I really appreciate if you want to leave your review. It's so important for me.

Manufactured by Amazon.ca
Bolton, ON

24578626R00092